Problematic Sexual Behavior in Schools

Problematic Sexual Behavior in Schools

How to Spot It and What to Do about It

Second Edition

J. Wilson Kenney

ROWMAN & LITTLEFIELD
Lanham • Boulder • New York • London

Published by Rowman & Littlefield
An imprint of The Rowman & Littlefield Publishing Group, Inc.
4501 Forbes Boulevard, Suite 200, Lanham, Maryland 20706
www.rowman.com

6 Tinworth Street, London SE11 5AL, United Kingdom

British Library Cataloguing in Publication Information Available

Library of Congress Cataloging-in-Publication Data
Names: Kenney, Wilson, 1972- author. | Kenney, Wilson, 1972- Sexual misconduct in
    children. | Rowman and Littlefield, Inc.
Title: Problematic sexual behavior in schools : how to spot it and what to do about it /
    J. Wilson Kenney.
Other titles: Sexual misconduct in children
Description: Second Edition. | Lanham : Rowman & Littlefield, 2020. | Originally
    published: Lanham : Rowman & Littlefield Education, 2013, by Wilson Kenney
    under title Sexual misconduct in children. | Includes bibliographical references. |
    Summary: "Problematic Sexual Behavior and Schools provides schools and
    communities all the information they need to establish a systematic approach for
    identifying and addressing problematic sexual behavior in children"— Provided by
    publisher.
Identifiers: LCCN 2020011077 (print) | LCCN 2020011078 (ebook) | ISBN
    9781475844375 (Cloth : acid-free paper) | ISBN 9781475844382 (Paperback :
    acid-free paper) | ISBN 9781475844399 (ePub)
Subjects: LCSH: Psychosexual disorders in children. | Children and sex. |
    Children—Sexual behavior. | Child sexual abuse—Prevention. | Child sex offenders.
Classification: LCC RJ506.P72 K46 2020 (print) | LCC RJ506.P72 (ebook) |
    DDC 618.92/8583—dc23
LC record available at https://lccn.loc.gov/2020011077
LC ebook record available at https://lccn.loc.gov/2020011078

This book is dedicated with love to my wife.
You are the main event of my life.

Contents

Preface

It became clear to me that an updated version of this book was needed for a few important reasons. The first reason had to do with the fact that some of the nomenclature around problematic sexual behavior had changed, which explains the change in the title of this book. *Sexual misconduct* was the term I used to refer to problematic sexual behavior in the first edition, and it's a term that is overly pathologizing and far too limiting. So, it's out, and *problematic sexual behavior*, which casts a wider and friendlier nomological net, is in.

An updated version was also needed because I had learned some new things that I thought might be useful. One of those I'll relay right now—problematic sexual behavior is behavior, first and foremost. It is important that we don't let our terror about the "problematic sexual" stuff make us forget what we already know: namely, that all behavior is communication that makes sense, given its context. Behavior is telling you a story. It's relaying something important. If we are curious and ask good questions, we can learn something valuable. Maintain your curiosity.

Another reason for a new edition of this book had to do with changes in our cultural context. We've benefited from some amazing paradigm shifts recently, like the Me Too Movement, which has helped to reorganize our thinking about sexual harassment and sexual assault. When I first wrote this book, some of the criticism I received was that I was pathologizing normative behavior by casting such a wide nomological net on problematic sexual behavior. Was it such a big deal if a kindergartener was touching the butt of a classmate? Should we really apply this method if a freshman kissed a female peer in the hallway after she told him not to? Isn't this all just normal kid behavior?

My thinking continues to be, we need to address all these forms of problematic sexual behavior. Some compelling research by Abbey and McAuslan

(A Longitudinal Examination of Male College Student Perpetration of Sexual Assault, 2004) indicates that individuals who engage in sexually assaultive behavior as adults exhibited misogynistic attitudes and engaged in sexually harassing behavior long before they started assaulting people sexually. So, in my mind, these problems start early and this methodological approach enables us to identify and change sexually problematic behavior when it is just starting to evidence itself, before sexual harm occurs. Simply put, we'd have a lot fewer adolescents and adults harming people sexually if we could do a better job of identifying and addressing these behaviors early on. So, cast a wide net. Be curious about all of it.

When I set out to get my doctorate in clinical psychology, I had no intention of ever working for a school district. My goal was to open up a little private practice and conduct forensic assessments on sexual offenders (SOs) (which is what I do now). I initially took a job as a school psychologist, however, because the pay and benefits were good, and because I had the opportunity to do plenty of evaluation. I had no idea when I started how much I would love working in public education, or that I would get involved in threat assessment.

In many respects, my work, and this book, is really the result of being the right guy, in the right place, at the right time. The district where I worked just happened to send me to a training session at Salem-Keizer Public Schools on their threat assessment system where I met John Van Dreal, the facilitator for the targeted threat response team for that district. We got to talking about gaps in that system, and specifically the need for a model that would address problematic sexual behavior. I told John about my background assessing youth with problematic sexual behavior, and within a year I was hired by that district to create a threat assessment system that would address problematic sexual behavior in schools. It was a dream job in an innovative district filled with smart and eager people.

This book is a detailed account of the system I developed while working at Salem-Keizer School District. The stories included herein are purely fictitious accounts I developed for the purpose of illustrating how to use the system. The names, histories, and details do not represent actual people or situations, and any resemblance they bear to actual events or actual people is purely coincidental. That being said, I tried my best to craft stories that accurately represent the kinds of situations one encounters when working in schools.

When I first started working at Salem-Keizer, I was uncertain how great a need there would be for a team that specifically addressed problematic sexual behavior. Initially, this model was considered to be sort of the younger brother to the targeted threat assessment team that was designed to identify potential school shooters. However, within a matter of months it became clear that administrators and school counselors were hungry for consultation in addressing sexual behavior in schools, and it wasn't long before I was receiving calls from public schools, private schools, and colleges all around the country seeking advice on what to do with these kids.

I was surprised. And in that state of shock I began to reconsider how the model for assessing problematic sexual behavior compared to the targeted (school shooter) threat assessment model. It dawned on me that, to some degree, the targeted threat assessment model was designed to find the proverbial needle in the haystack. It's a tool created to help identify that one in a million kid who is planning to harm others on a massive scale.

Some would say that the targeted threat assessment model is really just an insurance policy against the worst day of your life. The base rate suggests that it's very unlikely any particular district will contain a school shooter, but the costs for failing to correctly identify that potential school shooter are phenomenally high. Statistically speaking, you probably don't need a targeted threat assessment system for your district, but you cannot afford not to have it.

Regarding the assessment of problematic sexual behavior in schools, the model is just the opposite. Without question, there are a multitude of students in every district who are evidencing problems with regard to their sexual behavior. Some of these kids have very serious problems and may go on to harm others, some of these kids are being victimized and need rescuing, and some of these kids are just confused about what is appropriate and need direction. This is not like looking for the needle in the haystack; rather, problematic sexual behavior is the haystack.

In doing this work, I also came to learn how challenging and anxiety provoking it can be for the uninitiated. Most people don't enjoy talking about sexual behavior and this is even more evident when it comes to discussing the sexual behavior of children. Week after week, as I attended meetings, I saw the relief on the faces of the school counselors, administrators, and parents when they learned there was someone in the room who could help them talk about these difficult issues. I began to joke that if school administrators ever developed the ability to say "penis" without blushing, I'd be out of a job.

Silly, but true.

Parents, teachers, and administrators were deeply concerned about the sexual development and problematic sexual behavior of their children; they just didn't have a means for carrying on the dialogue and figuring out how best to proceed. There was fear, there was confusion, and there was anger. Really, more than anything, this book was written in order to help facilitate that dialogue. It's intended to assist concerned parties in cutting through the tension and getting to the two most important things: helping kids with problematic sexual behavior and protecting the community from harm.

I know that not every district can afford to bring on a specialist in problematic sexual behavior for consultation, and this book is intended to serve as the next best thing. It is my hope and my goal that this book will assist you in improving student and staff safety in your district. I believe that by implementing the practice in this book, you will be able to identify students with problematic sexual behavior sooner, intervene more effectively, and consequently decrease the impact of sexual harm in your school and community. A worthy goal if ever there was one.

Acknowledgments

I'd like to acknowledge several people who helped to make the second edition of this book possible. First and foremost, I want to thank my wife, Dr. Cassandra Kenney, who patiently helped me sculpt the ideas in this book and who was a compassionate and helpful editor. I'm a lucky man to have such an intelligent, supportive, and beautiful person as my partner.

I also owe a great debt to John Van Dreal, who, in addition to being a great friend and officiating my wedding (thanks again Johnny!), helped me land the job that enabled me to craft this model and also put me in touch with the publisher of this book. John also provided me permission to use the SIRC forms in this book (although it must be noted that they are outdated, as a new version was being developed around the same time this second edition was being drafted).

A special thanks to Marion County DDA's Brendan Murphy, JD, and David Wilson, JD, who both provided me ideas about interfacing with the DA's office via SIRC (their feedback is included in the Special Considerations chapter).

I'd also like to thank Mary Kane, JD, senior legal counsel for Portland Public Schools, and Liane O'Banion, EdD, Title IX director for Portland Public Schools, who wrote a chapter for this book on SIRC and Title IX. Last, but certainly not least, I'd like to thank Delaney Banas, PsyD, and Molly Persky, PsyD, who have patiently tolerated my ramblings and also generously contributed a chapter to this book.

Introduction

The bus driver had no idea it was going on. It's understandable. With those high-backed bus seats and the constant chaos, it's a challenge just to navigate the busy city streets. On the video, you can't really make out what exactly is happening in the third row up from the back of the bus. The tape is grainy. It's a little out of focus.

Sure, there were a few kids who might have seen something, first and second graders mostly. Not exactly what you'd call the best witnesses. There was a fourth grader behind them, kind of an odd kid, who had no idea what was going on just one seat ahead.

It's hard to say if anything actually happened at all. And even if what those two girls are claiming is true, how serious is it? Were they just playing around, or is it a problem? How am I supposed to know? And if it's a problem, what am I supposed to do about it?

Children's sexual behavior—a cringe-worthy topic if there ever was one. A topic guaranteed to strike fear into the boldest school counselor and leave the most battle-hardened administrator as goofy and red-faced as a preadolescent at their first dance. It's the one topic that causes grown-ups to spell out words like S-E-X and P-E-N-I-S, and it generally leaves most of us feeling foolish and "icky." Countless sitcoms have squeezed laughs out of the clichéd ineptitude of adults lamely attempting to discuss sexuality with regard to children. We all sit on the sidelines and laugh, but those who have had to broach this topic with a scared and angry parent, or query children about problematic sexual behavior, know that these clichés develop for a reason.

Aside from our general discomfort around discussing children's sexual behavior, it can be difficult to know what to make of these behaviors because there are so few resources that can help us make determinations about which behaviors are concerning and which behaviors are not. With no clear guidelines regarding sexual behavior in children, it becomes impossible to formulate a reasonable response, which can lead to making foolish fear-based decisions. No one wants to be the person who ignored problematic sexual behavior in a child, but no one wants to be the lead in a nationally syndicated news program after suspending a student over a seemingly minor infraction like kissing. Having a basic understanding of what is normative and nonnormative with regard to sexual behavior in children is essential to formulating a response. Consider the following:

> *Seth, assistant principal for a rural middle school, returned from a cabinet meeting to find, Maggie, the mother of one of his sixth grade girls, waiting to see him. Maggie's three children have all had their problems in school, but her youngest, Coleen, has been the most difficult child for her. According to Maggie, Coleen came back from a sleepover at her friend Janet's house acting very strangely.*
>
> *Essentially, Maggie spent the day badgering her daughter until Coleen eventually gave-in and reported that she had woken up suddenly during the sleepover and found Janet touching her "yoo-hoo." Maggie is convinced that Janet is a "pervert" and wants to know what Seth is going to do about it. As is typical for her in moments of stress, Maggie is beside herself with emotion and uncertain what to do about the situation.*

Is this behavior unusual for kids this age? Is Seth obligated to contact Child Protection Services? Should Seth interview Janet and attempt to get to the bottom of this on his own? What should he be doing to help Maggie? Is there a need for increased school supervision for these two girls, or should Seth ignore this because it happened outside of school? Without a basic playbook and a systematic method to guide his decision-making, Seth doesn't have much of a chance of dealing with this problem effectively.

Liz is an administrator of a small elementary school in a suburban area outside of a major city. A teacher at Liz's school informed her that he had caught two third-grade boys, John and Raymond, showing each other their "privates" during recess. The teacher was uncertain how to proceed and so he sent the boys to the principal's office. He also wasn't sure if he should complete a referral for the boys because he "didn't want to make a big deal out of it." Liz is uncertain how to proceed, but does her best to handle it as she would other behavioral issues: interview the boys separately, decide upon a disciplinary action, and call their parents.

Upon interviewing the boys, Liz is even less certain what to do. John, a popular boy who is big for his size and occasionally in trouble for bullying, seems largely unconcerned. He claims that Raymond walked up to him on the playground and showed him his penis. John denies provoking Raymond in any way, and he claims he has no idea why Raymond did it.

Raymond, a boy with few friends, is visibly shaken. He is initially quite tearful and insistent that Liz not call his dad. He neither confirms nor denies John's claims and says he doesn't want to talk about it. Liz decides to send John back to class and leaves Raymond sitting outside her office in the hopes that he will calm down.

Should Liz return John to class? What if John was the instigator? Why is Raymond so shaken up about such a little thing? Is Liz asking the right questions? Does Liz need to call law enforcement? Is this a big deal, or not?

Like most administrators faced with this sort of situation, Liz lacks the expertise to understand how best to proceed. She is uncertain what occurred, she doesn't know what questions to ask, and even if she did, she wouldn't know what to do with the information.

To further complicate the situation, Liz is expected to assume the weight and legal liability of making this decision largely by herself. Sure, she can consult with her level directors, or beg the advice of her school counselor, but her resources suffer from the same problem. They don't know any more than Liz about problematic sexual behavior in kids and they don't understand how to manage it any better than she does.

Six weeks into the first semester, Kelly, Freshman counselor at a large urban high school, finally received the file on Brian, a mainstream, out-of-state transfer. She wouldn't have time to read through it now, but she guessed from its weight that Brian was a very complicated student. Kelly hustled toward her administrator's office, with Brian's file tucked under her arm.

During the meeting with her administrator, Kelly learns that Brian has been evidencing serious behavior problems for the last three weeks. He makes strange sexual sounds in class, tries to wipe his snot on his classmates, and frequently puts his hand down the back of his pants in class. Today, Brian was discovered sexually harassing a female classmate.

According to the female student, Brian cornered her during their early childcare class, a class where high school students get hands-on experience working in the on-site daycare, and told her he was going to "follow her home and rape her." He then waved his finger under her nose, which she claimed "smelled disgusting. I almost threw up." The administrator suspended Brian for five days, so that he and Kelly can figure out what to do about him.

How serious is Brian's threat? Should the administrator have suspended Brian? Is the female student he harassed in any danger? What about the children in early childcare? Should law enforcement be involved? Are there any liability or safety concerns that extend beyond the campus? Is there anyone Kelly can consult with to figure out what to do about this?

Like most school counselors, Kelly wants to make sure that Brian gets the help he needs and she wants to make sure that students at school are safe. She's just not sure exactly how to make those two things happen simultaneously.

WHAT IS NEEDED?

In order for these decision makers to effectively handle these problems, they need four things: (1) to know the most important questions to ask, and how to ask them, (2) a basic understanding of what is developmentally normative and nonnormative sexual behavior for children, (3) a systematic means for addressing safety and supervision and handling liability, and (4) a method for accessing expertise and community support when additional help is needed.

Knowing the right questions to ask, and having the proper language to discuss a situation helps decision makers gather the information they need to make good decisions, and it communicates a level of expertise and professionalism that helps parents feel more confident and less afraid in a stressful situation. Having basic knowledge about what kinds of sexual behavior to expect among children as a function of their development can help decision makers determine how serious a situation is and provide some early clues for how best to handle the situation. Possessing a systematic method for addressing safety, supervision, and liability insures that potentially dangerous situations get handled in a consistent manner that is in line with best practice, rather than individual subjective judgment. Finally, having a means to access expertise and community support when needed ensures that even the most complicated situations will be addressed appropriately and professionally, thereby improving community safety and limiting exposure to liability.

Crafting a system that provides all this may at first appear like a Herculean task, but it's not. In fact, these goals can be accomplished by (1) developing a few protocols (examples of which you will see in the appendices), (2) doing a few hours of training each year (on information I've included in this book), (3) formalizing and adopting a strategy for examining problematic sexual behavior (which is outlined in this book), and (4) creating a multiagency team to provide expertise and support (similar to Youth Service Teams that likely already exist in your region and which is, yes you guessed it, also outlined in this book).

This book will teach you the important questions to ask when addressing problematic sexual behavior, it will provide you with the language to discuss these difficult issues with confidence, and it will help you to understand the differences between normative and nonnormative sexual behavior in children. This book will also provide insights into addressing the liability that exists around educating kids with potentially harmful sexual behavior, and it will provide real-world, budget-conscious strategies for providing excellent supervision and intervention. You will also find a number of helpful forms at the back of this book (in the appendixes) you can adapt to help you in your endeavor. In short, this book will remove the fear and uncertainty you currently experience when problematic sexual behaviors come across your desk, and provide you a systematic methodology for handling even the toughest situations.

Chapter 1

Threat Assessment

A Brief History Lesson

In order to understand and justify the system outlined in this book, it is important to first have an understanding of where threat assessment has been and how it got here. Prior to the "epidemic" of school shootings that occurred in the mid-1990s, threat assessment was mostly the business of psychologists, psychiatrists, and federal law enforcement officials.

In that "pre-Columbine" era, the term *threat assessment* typically referred to some type of process designed to help professionals make a prediction regarding the likelihood that an individual would commit a future harmful sexual or violent act. In most cases, that process involved a single threat assessment professional administering a battery of psychological tests to the individual of concern, conducting a careful examination of their history, and interviewing them on a host of topics, after which the professional would produce a report indicating the risk for harm to others and, ideally, the conditions under which the individual was most likely to act in a harmful way.

The approach to threat assessment in those earlier days was not unlike the method biologists employ when examining biological life in a pond, and in fact, this was a common metaphor used to help laymen understand the utility of assessment. According to this notion, the threat assessment evaluator was thought to be "sampling the pond water" when they conducted an evaluation, essentially "dipping a ladle" into the subject's psyche and "examining the contents under a microscope" in order to make a determination about "the contents of the pond," in this case, a person's potential to harm others.

In spite of their best intentions, however, the fact is, this is not really what threat assessment professionals were doing. In truth, threat assessment professionals were in disagreement about how exactly to sample the pond water, how to analyze its contents, and what the contents suggested about the pond in general.

Additionally, these professionals were unintentionally but routinely putting a number of other things in the pond water that impacted the results of the assessment (i.e., their own bias), and they were failing to include very important elements such as what was occurring outside the pond (i.e., context). As a result of these inconsistencies, it became very difficult to ascertain what exactly was being assessed in a threat assessment and how relevant the findings were to predicting threat.

One of the biggest problems, however, with this method of conducting threat assessments was that the underlying "pond water" theory was completely misguided. Although there is generous evidence to support the notion that many aspects of our personality and psychology are relatively stable (like pond water), there is also abundant evidence that just as many aspects are changeable and adaptable. This suggests that the human psyche is as much like a stream as it is a pond. And therein, more than anywhere, lies the rub. Although a ladle full of pond water may contain an abundance of useful information regarding the overall contents of the pond, the same cannot be said about a ladle full of ever-changing stream water, whose contents generally reveal very little about the entire stream beyond that brief moment of extraction at that particular point in the stream.

This is not to suggest that traditional threat assessment has no value. It can still be very helpful to consider aspects of the psyche when attempting to predict future harmful behavior. Rather, this line of reasoning suggests that the value and scope of traditional threat assessment is very limited, because it fails to consider three very important areas: assessor bias, the passage of time, and environmental influences (i.e., context).

Human beings are ridiculously prone to bias. We oftentimes make decisions based upon our gut, and as repeatedly demonstrated in scientific study, we tend to stick with those decisions even when presented with conflicting evidence. The more we argue for or defend our opinions, the more likely we are to believe them, even when those opinions are challenged with irrefutable evidence.

When it comes to threat assessment, bias can lead us to misperceive the seriousness of threat, giving a dangerous psychopath a second chance to harm others or potentially burning an innocent at the stake. When we leave the responsibility of determining threat to a single individual or assessment process, we increase the likelihood that the results of that assessment reflect, at least in part, bias on the part of the evaluator. Ideally, to prevent bias, threat assessment should incorporate the opinions and assessments of multiple individuals from multidisciplinary perspectives. More about that later.

It is not a secret that traditional threat assessment does an abysmal job dealing with the passage of time. Generally speaking, traditional threat assessments take weeks to months to produce. In highly volatile situations, when harmful behavior is on the table, supervision agencies like schools and probation agencies do not have the luxury of time that it takes to produce traditional threat assessments. They need answers right away, and they need a comprehensive supervision plan they can put into place immediately.

Supervision agencies also need information that is timely and relevant, which is impossible for traditional threat assessment to provide. In fact, any decent traditional threat assessment report will boldly state that the results of that assessment cannot account for the passage of time, and that the report itself has an expiration date. This is problematic because threatening situations improve or worsen with the passage time (sometimes very quickly), as various interventions are employed and as the individual and his or her environment change. It is too costly and time consuming to conduct multiple traditional threat assessments in an attempt to keep pace with the ever-changing stream. Ultimately, what is needed is a means of quickly and cheaply assessing an individual on an ongoing basis. More about that later too.

Traditional threat assessment's failure to include important environmental factors and contextual information, however, is likely the biggest problem with this method of assessment. In a careful examination of school shootings that was conducted by the Secret Service, one of the most important findings was that the biggest problem with identifying and predicting threat (at least violent threat) was not lack of information, but poor communication between educational, mental health, and law enforcement agencies.

In other words, when it came to school shootings, there was abundant information that threatening behavior was imminent, but that information was not getting shared between stakeholders. Each agency had a piece of the puzzle, but there was no means of putting all those pieces together in order to see the big picture.

Although, this discovery was based upon an examination of school shootings, there is cause to believe that employing a strategy that enables multiple agencies to discuss concerning threatening behavior, violent or sexual, improves the assessment of threat. Agencies don't necessarily need to become better at extracting information, rather they need to become more proficient at sharing information with other agencies. You guessed it—more about that later as well.

What is needed is a cheap, easy, and quick mechanism for gathering real-time threat-specific data from multiple sources, sharing that data in a timely fashion, and crafting a timely helpful response that is less prone to bias than traditional threat assessment. The mechanism to accomplish all this is to adopt a leveled sexual behavior assessment system similar to the leveled threat assessment systems that have been successfully protecting our schools and communities from violent threats for over two decades.

THE LEVELED THREAT ASSESSMENT SYSTEM

The two-level system is a mechanism for gathering and sharing time-sensitive, risk-specific information. The model was initially developed by the Secret Service as a means for anticipating and addressing threatening and violent behavior. Although the system was created for the purpose of identifying potential school shooters, the basic mechanics of this approach work just as well with regard to addressing other forms of threatening behavior including problematic sexual behavior.

Here's how it works:

1. School officials learn that problematic sexual behavior or the threat of problematic sexual behavior has occurred on or off school grounds, before, during, or after school and file a report with the appropriate protective body (i.e., law enforcement, Child Protective Services, or the Department of Human Services [DHS]).

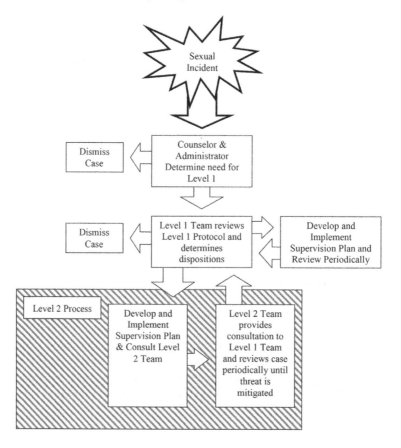

2. School administrator and school counselor make the decision to either conduct a Level 1 examination or dismiss the case.
3. School administrator and school counselor immediately convene a Level 1 team meeting and answer the questions in the Level 1 protocol.
4. Based upon the results of the Level 1 protocol, the Level 1 team decides to dismiss the case or develop a supervision plan and/or request a Level 2 team review if additional consultation is required.
5. In the event that a Level 2 consultation is sought out, the Level 2 team (a multiagency/multidisciplinary team that meets on a weekly basis to offer consultation and resources to Level 1 teams) convenes, reviews the details of the case and provides immediate feedback to the Level 1 team. The Level 2 team continues to follow cases until they are resolved to the satisfaction of the Level 2 team and the risk is effectively mitigated.

Let's take each step and look at it more closely. Step 1: School officials learn that an incident of problematic sexual behavior has occurred. It doesn't matter where or when that event occurred (or even if it actually occurred at all) because once you have the reasonable suspicion that some problematic sexual behavior has occurred, you also have the liability for failing to respond to that information appropriately.

In step 1, you need to document that a case of problematic sexual behavior was alleged, typically via a behavioral referral, progress note and/or child welfare notification documentation (i.e., from law enforcement, Child Protective Services, and/or DHS). This information should go into a specially marked confidential file folder that is stored in the student's academic record. It is wise to limit staff access to this file such that it should only be read by administrators, school counselors, and individuals to whom the administrator has given direct permission.

The most frequently asked question about documentation is, "do I document and report every little thing . . . even when I catch six-year-old Billy peeing in the barkdust?" Generally, it's wise to err on the side of caution. It's likely that Billy peeing in the barkdust is just a function of his not yet being socialized for the school experience, but it's also possible that something more concerning may be afoot. Protective agencies vary widely with regard to the types of incidents that they consider reportable, and so school officials need to work closely with protective agencies in their area to determine what the threshold should be for reportable incidents.

From a risk and liability mitigation perspective, however, every concerning behavior needs to be documented in some fashion. That does not suggest that every concerning behavior needs to be addressed immediately, and it certainly doesn't suggest that you conduct a comprehensive assessment (or Level 1) for every problem you encounter. But it is important to, at the very least, document what is occurring because that information helps you and your team track behaviors that are of a concern to you. Maybe that first incident of peeing in the barkdust is not a big deal, but when it's happened for the tenth time, you'll be wishing you had documented all those occurrences.

Step 2: The administrator of record and the school counselor meet to determine if the situation warrants a Level 1 team meeting. A Level 1 team meeting should be recommended if any of the following criteria are met:

1. The student's sexual behavior is causing disruption in school or community activities (i.e., staff, parents, or peers perceive the sexual incident as bothersome, unusual, odd, or inappropriate).
2. Interventions designed to decrease the problematic sexual behavior have been unsuccessful.
3. There is a history of sexually inappropriate behavior.
4. The administrator and school counselor are unable to assert that the concern is unfounded.

Whether or not to conduct a Level 1 team meeting is always the toughest call in elementary schools and with cognitively impaired students. No one has any questions about whether or not it's concerning when a seventh-grade student is caught rubbing his or her genitals against a desk or a teacher's leg, but it's much less clear when a first grader engages in this behavior. It's obvious that high school age students should not be exposing their genitals to their peers, but it's hard to determine how serious the behavior is when that student has an IQ below seventy.

Any eighth grader caught masturbating in class will undoubtedly receive a few days of suspension, but should a kindergartener or a cognitively impaired student be treated the same? You don't want to create a situation where you are conducting a Level 1 meeting every other day over minor indiscretions, but you also don't want to ignore a serious problem that is bubbling to the surface. Making the call on younger or cognitively impacted students can be difficult, but applying the criteria listed above can be very helpful. Let's take a moment to explore those criteria in more detail.

DISRUPTION

Is the behavior causing disruption? Odds are that you are going to start receiving complaints from staff, students, and parents if the problematic sexual behavior is disruptive to school. If the teacher can't get through basic instruction because the problematic sexual behavior is so disruptive, or the student's peers are starting to discuss the behavior, or parents are calling the school about it, then it likely warrants a Level 1 meeting.

RESPONSIVE TO INTERVENTION

Does the behavior respond to intervention? Sexual behavior that does not respond to intervention should be taken very seriously. Generally speaking, most children don't enjoy adults talking to them about their sexual behavior. If you've had a talk with the student and his or her parents, and tried some behavioral interventions to inhibit the problematic sexual behavior, and yet the behavior persists, you probably need to take it to a Level 1 team meeting.

Keep in mind that although not every situation warrants a call to law enforcement or a Level 1 meeting, every situation does require a meaningful and appropriate response of some kind. You don't need to conduct a Level 1 when you catch seven-year-old Billy peeing in the barkdust, or eight-year-old Suzie rubbing her genitals against the side of her desk. But you do need to document this behavior, and it would be wise to engage in some type of intervention designed to decrease the behavior. In most situations, a call home or a small intervention is all that is needed to turn the behavior around. If your attempts fail, then you can always turn to Level 1.

HISTORY

Does the student have a history of problematic sexual behavior? When it comes to problematic sexual behavior, the best predictor of future behavior is past behavior. If the student has a history of acting out sexually, then you probably want to schedule a Level 1 meeting immediately.

UNCERTAINTY

Finally, if you can't determine that a concern doesn't exist, go ahead with a Level 1 meeting. At the very least, the Level 1 meeting is a great mechanism for confidently dismissing a concern.

THE LEVEL 1

Okay. You've decided you can't dismiss the concern and you need to conduct a Level 1 meeting. Time is of the essence and it's ideal if you can conduct the meeting on the same day that you learn about the behavior.

The purpose of this meeting is so that the school can make a determination about how to proceed about the problematic sexual behavior. Although this meeting is really about making sure that students are safe and that students with problematic sexual behavior get help, you must also bear in mind that this meeting is also about addressing liability at the school. Consequently, the only people who need to be in attendance and review the Level 1 protocol are the administrator of record and the school counselor.

Remember, a Level 1 meeting is not a disciplinary mechanism. If the student needs to have school discipline for his or her problematic sexual behavior, it should be handled via a separate meeting consistent with your district's disciplinary protocols.

Although only the administrator and counselor need to be in attendance at a Level 1 meeting, it is recommended that you also invite the student's parents and any other collaterals who might be useful in making a determination regarding the seriousness of the student's behavior and/or helpful in developing a supervision plan. Those collaterals might include the student's legal guardian, law enforcement/school resource officer, DHS case worker, Court Appointed Special Advocate (CASA), parole/probation officer, foster parent, special education (SPED) case manager, and so on.

Level 1 meetings don't generally need to include a student's classroom teacher unless you have reason to believe that the classroom teacher might have particular insight into the nature of the problematic sexual behavior. However, if the student is a SPED student, it's important to have their SPED or 504 case manager in attendance to ensure that the supervision decisions you make do not impact the Individualized Education or 504 Plan. In the event that potential team members cannot attend the Level 1 meeting, they can be encouraged to provide feedback via phone or via a semi-structured interview (you can find a copy of this in appendix B) designed to gather information for the Level 1 protocol.

During the Level 1 meeting, the team will complete the Level 1 protocol (you can find a copy of this in appendix A) and determine how best to triage the case. The Level 1 team may decide to (a) dismiss the case, (b) develop and implement a supervision plan and review its implementation periodically, or (c) develop and implement a supervision plan and request Level 2 consultation.

In the event that the case is dismissed by the Level 1 team, the decision to dismiss is recorded in the Level 1 protocol, which is then filed in the confidential file folder in the student's academic record. If the team decides to develop and implement a supervision plan, this is recorded in the Level 1 protocol (which is filed in the confidential file folder in the student's academic record). The protocol is periodically reviewed by the supervision team members to ensure fidelity to the supervision plan, and determine how best to adjust the plan to meet the student's supervision needs.

Should the team decide to request Level 2 consultation, a copy of the Level 1 protocol is sent to the Level 2 team. The preliminary supervision plan is recorded in the Level 1 protocol, which is filed in the confidential file folder in the student's academic record (sensing a pattern yet?), and this preliminary plan is followed until the Level 2 team communicates recommendations to the Level 1 team, at which point the supervision plan is updated to reflect these recommendations.

THE LEVEL 2

Once a Level 2 consultation is requested, the facilitator of the Level 2 team contacts the Level 1 team and immediately schedules time to meet with the school counselor and/or administrator to gather additional information, prior to the Level 2 meeting. During this information gathering, or Level 2 inquiry, the facilitator gathers background information on the student to assist the Level 2 team in providing consultation. After this meeting occurs, the Level 2 facilitator shares the gathered data and the Level 1 referral with the Level 2 team.

The Level 2 team is a multidisciplinary/multiagency team that meets on a regular basis to discuss problematic sexual incidents and provide consultation to schools and community partners regarding the supervision and intervention of students with problematic sexual behavior. During the Level 2 meeting, the Level 2 facilitator shares the details of the case and encourages discussion regarding how best to respond to and manage the sexual behavior.

The Level 2 team provides their recommendations back to the Level 1 team, who then choose which recommendations they intend to implement. The Level 2 team then continues to track the progress of the Level 1 referral through regular check-ins with the Level 1 team, until the behavior is considered by both the Level 1 and Level 2 teams to be successfully managed. At which point the case is retired.

WHY THIS IS SO COOL

There are a number of wonderful things about the leveled threat response system. First and foremost, it's very fast. Gone are the days of waiting weeks or months for a threat assessment or psychosexual evaluation. By employing this system, you will be able to respond to problematic sexual behavior on the day it occurs and receive meaningful consultation immediately.

Second, this model is incredibly responsive to changes with regard to the seriousness of the threat, because the assessment and intervention are dynamic and continuous. Further, because the intervention and supervision strategies are developed and monitored via ongoing communication between the Level 1 team (who has their feet on the ground) and the Level 2 team (who has access to all the expertise), you have the capacity to constantly keep your finger on the pulse with regard to safety and risk mitigation. If the student's behavior is worsening, you have the ability to assess the potential threat on the day it occurs, and you have the capacity to respond immediately. Conversely, if the student's behavior improves and you have good cause to believe that the potential threat has decreased (say you have a letter from his or her therapist stating that risk has been reduced), you can also respond to that immediately.

Another advantage of this system is that it is much less prone to bias than relying upon traditional means. By using the Level 1 system, you are systematizing your approach to addressing problematic sexual behavior and reducing the likelihood that your decision-making is based on gut. Everyone in your district uses the same Level 1 protocol, which means that the results are likely to be more consistent from one administrator to another.

In those instances when a Level 1 team feels out of their depth, administrators can consult with a multiagency team of professionals via the Level 2 process. That Level 2 team is also less prone to individual bias in their planning and intervention recommendations because they function as a multidisciplinary team rather than as a single individual.

Finally, one of the biggest advantages of this model for assessing threat is its capacity to consider context. Level 2 teams have the advantage of operating with the "big picture," one that includes not only the school, but the community at large, and receives input from law enforcement, Department of Juvenile Justice, DHS and other community partners.

A NOTE ABOUT LIABILITY

Imagine the following scenarios. Derek is a father of two little girls, ages eight and six. His eight-year-old, Leslie, recently reported that an older boy at school touched her vagina during recess. Derek, like any reasonable father, calls the classroom teacher to ascertain what happened. During his phone call, Derek learns that Leslie and a few of her classmates have been complaining about being harassed by the boy Leslie mentioned. The classroom teacher indicates that she will call in a report to DHS and refers Derek to the school counselor for further discussion. The next day Leslie returns to school and is again sexually assaulted by the boy who touched her vagina the day before.

Rebecca is a school counselor. Monday morning, she receives a call from Mary, an upset mother of two. Mary reports that over the weekend, her son Craig was sexually molested by a fellow classmate, Charlie, while on a sleepover at a friend's house. Rebecca does her best to soothe and calm Mary, offers her a phone number to a local therapist, and after concluding the call contacts law enforcement to report the allegation. Two days later, a teacher hears crying in the boy's bathroom and discovers Charlie attempting to anally penetrate Craig in a restroom stall.

Peter has a well-documented history of problematic sexual behavior and is on a safety plan that was developed by the school administrator and school counselor, neither of whom know much about problematic sexual behavior. Because Peter has been doing such a good job academically, the school administrator decides to loosen the supervision plan. Two days after doing this, Peter sexually assaults a cognitively disabled girl while she is attempting to use the restroom.

Chris is a new high school student who has been evidencing some serious behavioral problems and blowing off his academic classes. In an attempt to lighten his workload, while the staff gets to know him, Chris was placed in the childcare class because he reported he likes working with children. After two days in the classroom, Chris is caught sexually touching one of the toddlers and is immediately reported to law enforcement. Upon reviewing Chris's transfer file a week later, the school counselor discovers a safety plan that was completed by his last school placement indicating that he should never be left alone with children because he has a history of sexually inappropriate behavior.

Each of these scenarios demonstrates common ways of addressing problematic sexual behavior that fail to adequately handle the problem, and ultimately leave the district exposed to tremendous liability. When these cases end up in litigation, it won't matter that the school counselor reported the case to authorities, that the school administrator didn't realize that reducing a safety plan on the basis of academic performance flies in the face of what is known about supervising kids with problematic sexual behavior, or that the school counselor didn't have time to read the whole file before putting Chris in the childcare class. As far as the courts are concerned, knowledge equals responsibility.

The leveled threat assessment is the best means for addressing liability concerns because it does two things. First, it operationalizes and mechanizes your approach to considering problematic sexual behavior, thereby improving the reliability and consistency of the decisions made by your Level 1 teams. What this means is that everyone who uses this approach (i.e., the Level 1 protocol) will be thinking about problematic sexual behavior in a very similar way, and that the conclusions they draw will be much more consistent than what would occur without such a system. Implementing this approach district wide means that, provided a school administrator follows the Level 1 protocol, she or he can feel confident that the way in which the case was handled was consistent with school policy and consequently more defensible in court.

The second way in which this model protects the district from liability is via the Level 2 team. Should the administrator or Level 1 team encounter a case of unusual complexity, the Level 2 team is there to provide consultation. Every recommendation made by the Level 2 team is made by a multidisciplinary/multiagency team. Consequently, the liability surrounding these decisions is spread across these agencies rather than assumed by a single school administrator, as is typically the case.

DOING WHAT IS BEST FOR KIDS

There is one final reason to adopt the leveled threat assessment approach. It's odd to save it for last, because it is probably the most important reason.

Having a leveled threat assessment system is best for kids and families. Because of its responsiveness and comprehensiveness, this is the best approach for protecting children, school staff, and your community from sexual harm. Because of its sensitivity to language and context, there is no better way to put families at ease and reassure them that the school has the expertise to handle these delicate problems. Finally, because of the thoughtfulness and care that went into crafting this approach, it is the best means of protecting the reputation of kids who are struggling with problematic sexual behavior, and getting them immediate access to the help and supervision they need so that they can become restored and avoid harming others.

Chapter 2

Problematic Sexual Behavior in Schools

Delaney Banas and Molly Persky

In order to address problematic sexual behavior in schools, it is important to understand the framework of what is known. Delaney Banas, PsyD, and Molly Persky, PsyD, generously offered this chapter to help put problematic sexual behavior in children in context.

It is something that no parent, teacher, or school administrator likes to think about: problematic sexual behavior among children. It is easy to take the perspective of "that won't happen here," or "kids don't even know what sex is." However, the reality is that problematic sexual behavior is occurring more than adults like to think about. Although the numbers may seem staggering, information that we *do* know about problematic sexual behavior in schools is likely a gross underestimation, due to several factors. There are ways to address these behaviors, most notably with proper supervision and treatment. This chapter focuses on what we know about problematic sexual behavior in schools, present difficulties in addressing sexual behavior in schools, and ways to address the problems through proper treatment and supervision,

WHAT DO WE KNOW?

The Associated Press (AP) conducted an in-depth investigation of problematic sexual behavior in schools over a four-year period (2011–2015). Please see https://www.ap.org/explore/schoolhouse-sex-assault/index.html for additional information. During this time, they found 17,000 official reports of problematic sexual behavior by students in U.S. elementary and secondary schools, making schools the second most common location for problematic sexual behavior following the home. Within schools, problematic sexual behavior typically occurs in areas with little to no supervision: buses, bathrooms, hallways, and locker rooms, for example. Although unwanted fondling was the most commonly reported type of incident, the severity of the reported behavior varied significantly. Across the incidents, one in five reported rape, sodomy, or penetration by an object.

So, who is engaging in this behavior, and why? Identification of potential perpetrators of problematic sexual behavior for the purpose of early intervention is difficult, as there is no "typical perpetrator" with regard to personality, background, or motivation for offending behavior. However, motivation appears to follow general trends with regard to age. In elementary school, most kids who engage in sexually inappropriate behavior appear motivated by sexual curiosity and ignorance about personal boundaries. In middle school, offenses seem to be driven by impulsivity and opportunity. In high school, offenses appear more closely related to feelings of entitlement and a desire to exert control over the victim.

The AP investigation noted that 5 percent of the reported problematic sexual behavior occurred with students between the ages of five and six. Incidents increased with students around age ten and continued to increase until age fourteen, and then decreased with the progression through high school. As young children, boys make up 41 percent of the victims, as opposed to only 10 percent of victims during adolescence. Most assaults occur between same-age peers. However, younger kids may also be the victim of older perpetrators, as the older children typically have more power (both social and physical), as well as increased knowledge.

As mentioned before, the available information is likely a gross underestimation of actual problematic sexual behavior. In a survey of state education departments conducted by the AP, only thirty-two states and the District of Columbia track student problematic sexual behavior. Some of these states only tracked an incident if it led to suspension or expulsion, and some of the nation's largest school districts reported zero problematic sexual behavior over a multiyear period, which seems at the very least unlikely, if not impossible. In 2014, the White House created a task force on student problematic sexual behavior and launched a website with prevention strategies and legal advice. Awareness of the campaign seemed successful, with the number of complaints increasing fourfold between 2014 and 2016.

DIFFICULTIES IN ADDRESSING THE PROBLEM

With the information described above, one might think problematic sexual behavior would be on the forefront of problems to be addressed within our school systems. However, problematic sexual behavior is an incredibly complex problem, and incomplete information makes incidents of problematic sexual behavior difficult to investigate. To begin, incidents are often underreported or reported substantially after the fact, at which time physical evidence rarely remains. As these incidents typically occur in areas of no supervision with few or no eyewitnesses, investigations typically devolve into a "he said, she said" situation in which administrators are reluctant to take disciplinary action or contact law enforcement without "concrete" evidence in either direction.

Furthermore, sexual incidents can be mislabeled as bullying, hazing, or consensual behavior. This is especially relevant within the context of organized sports, shown in the AP investigation to be the leading context for student-on-student sexual violence. Oftentimes, coaches may treat problematic sexual behavior as a team disciplinary manner rather than an incident needing legal or administrative intervention. In turn, the behaviors may persist or become cyclical, with the victims then becoming offenders trying to "one up" what was done to them by engaging in more severe or violent behavior. Victims may be especially reluctant to disclose abuse in these situations, fearing "rocking the boat." In some situations, there can be more backlash against victims, with the community supporting the coaches or the accused players.

Finally, broader systemic problems as well as a lack of legislation requiring tracking of problematic sexual behavior further complicates the ability to adequately address the problem. Probably to no surprise, schools with inadequate funding suffer with regard to resources for proper supervision and education. In contrast to college-level institutions, elementary and secondary schools have no national requirement to track or disclose sexual violence, solely recommendations provided by the U.S. Department of Education. In fact, there is oftentimes pressure to keep incidents of sexual violence well hidden, and schools may limit information provided about offenses in order to protect the accused students or the image of the school. As noted by Dr. Bill Howe during the AP investigation, "No principal wants to be the rape school." Finally, privacy laws often prevent offenders from being known within the school setting, impacting the ability for adequate supervision.

Problematic sexual behavior may seem like a daunting task to confront. For starters, we have an incomplete picture of the problem due to the aforementioned difficulties in reporting and subsequent tracking of incidents. Systemic factors further impact the ability to address problematic incidents. However, there is hope! General supervision and education, as well as treatment following incidents of problematic sexual behavior offer ways in which to hopefully increase the safety of school and decrease these incidents. The remainder of the chapter focuses on supervision and treatment strategies targeting problematic sexual behavior.

Is Sexual Offender Treatment Effective?

A long-held debate concerns whether SO treatment is effective at reducing the recidivism risk of SOs (Hanson et al., 2009). Several research studies have been conducted to address this question; however, the results are mixed. Perhaps the largest study conducted found that SO treatment was more effective at reducing recidivism rates of adult SOs when compared to no treatment (Schmucker & Lösel, 2008). The authors of this study also found that cognitive-behavioral programs were more effective at reducing recidivism than were other psychosocial approaches.

So, what makes SO treatment programs effective? Researchers have determined that adherence to a risk, need, and responsivity (RNR) model of treatment can significantly reduce the rates of recidivism in adult offenders (Hanson et al., 2009). In other words, treatments are effective when they treat offenders at greater risk, when they target specific characteristics related to reoffending, and when they match the treatment to the offenders' abilities and learning styles.

What does an RNR model of treatment look like for adults with sexual offenses? Hanson et al. (2009) examined a number of studies and meta-analysis to determine the extent to which treatment programs adhered to the RNR model of treatment. Programs that adhered to the "risk" principal provided "intensive interventions to higher risk offenders and little or no service to low risk offenders" (p. 871). Programs that adhered to the "need" principal utilized treatment targets that were related to sexual or general recidivism. Specifically, these treatments focused on criminogenic factors such as deviant sexual interests, sexual preoccupation, attitudes tolerant of sexual crime, and intimacy deficits. Finally, programs that adhered to the "responsivity" principal provided treatment in a manner that matched the learning style of the clients.

Overall, Hanson et al. (2009) found that evidence supporting the utilization of RNR principles was sufficient such that RNR should be a "primary consideration in the design and implementation of intervention programs for sexual offenders" (p. 886). The authors noted that most contemporary programs conform to some aspects of the responsivity principle, particularly cognitive-behavioral therapy approaches. However, they found that "attention to the need principle would motivate the largest changes in the interventions currently given to sexual offenders" (p. 886). Overall, although treatment has been shown to be effective, specific areas to be addressed seem largely unknown. For example, many of the factors typically targeted in contemporary treatment programs include offense responsibility, social skills training, and victim empathy. However, none of these variables have been found to predict sexual recidivism.

SO Treatment for Juveniles

Given what we know about SO treatment for adults, can we apply those same principles to juvenile sex offender (JSO) treatment? In the past, JSO treatment programs have primarily been modeled on adult SO treatment programs. However, research has emerged that indicates that juvenile and adult offenders differ in their development, motivation, and behavior. For example, juvenile offenders have been found to be more impulsive and less aware of the consequences of their actions than are adult offenders. As a result, JSO treatment programs are designed to address those behaviors. Further, these programs also take into account psychosocial factors such as families and peers (Przybylski, 2014). Part of the reason we can be more hopeful with JSO treatment is that so much of a juvenile's success in these programs revolves around the family system's influence.

Take for example two different cases involving sexual violence. The first case involves a thirty-five-year-old, single, adult male who sexually assaults a young female. He has no history of steady employment, no ties to the community, and no family members. What factors are likely to motivate him to reduce his sexual behavior, other than the threat of incarceration? Now let's examine the same sexual assault, however this time, the offender is a thirteen-year-old boy in the ninth grade. He lives at home with his two parents and younger sibling. What factors are likely to motivate him to reduce his sexual behavior? Although he will be influenced by the threat of incarceration, he is more likely to be influenced by his parents, his siblings, and his loved ones. The question remains though: are these programs effective?

A study was conducted in 2006 to determine the effectiveness of SO treatment for juveniles (Reitzel & Carbonell, 2006). In the study, the authors examined data from nine published and unpublished studies on juvenile offender treatment effectiveness in regard to recidivism. The authors found that, overall, the average rates of recidivism for sexual crimes among juveniles was 12.53 percent as compared to rates of nonsexual recidivism, which ranged from 20.40 percent (other/unspecified, nonsexual recidivism) to 28.51 percent (nonviolent, nonsexual recidivism). After examining the studies, the authors found that the results were consistent with research on juvenile and adult samples of treated offenders, such that lower recidivism rates were reported in treated juveniles when compared to treated adult offenders. Specifically, the authors found that offenders who received SO treatment had lower rates of sexual recidivism (7.4 percent) as compared to those receiving no treatment (18.9 percent). The authors also found that for every forty-three SOs who recidivated after having received JSO treatment, one hundred SOs receiving comparison treatment or no treatment recidivated. Thus, JSO treatment was found to be more effective at reducing recidivism rates of juvenile offenders than was comparison treatment or no treatment at all.

TYPES OF TREATMENT PROGRAMS

A variety of treatment programs have been developed to address the unique needs of juvenile SOs. For example, cognitive-behavioral therapy treatment programs have been found to be effective in helping juvenile offenders reduce their maladaptive thinking and engage in more pro-social behaviors (Rosner, 2003). A similar type of program, Cognitive-Behavioral Therapy/ Relapse Prevention (CBT-RP) involves helping the juvenile to identify high-risk situations and maladaptive thought patterns to develop methods for coping with, and understanding, their cycle of sexual abuse (Rosner, 2003); however, research is limited regarding its effectiveness for reducing JSO behavior (Letourneau & Borduin, 2008). Another approach to working with juvenile SOs is family systems therapy. This type of therapy uses a five-stage model to identify and interrupt the family patterns that contributed to the atypical sexual behavior. Further, the goal of this type of therapy is to improve family relationships and utilize the family as a support system for the juvenile (Rosner, 2003).

Other types of treatment programs include psychotherapeutic programs, which involve more traditional "talk-therapy" approaches. Such programs tend to target trauma related to the sexual abuse cycle. Multisystemic therapy is another approach to working with juvenile SOs (Letourneau et al., 2009). This approach targets the underlying sexual behavior by addressing the juveniles social and interpersonal interactions and by treating the offender within their environment (e.g., home, school).

Overall, there are a variety of therapeutic modalities to use when working with juvenile SOs. It's important to note that there is no "one-size-fits-all" approach. When deciding on a specific therapeutic modality, consideration must be made to psychosocial factors including resources, parental involvement, financial costs, and cultural factors.

WHAT ARE THE NUMBERS?

In a district of roughly 40,000 kids (the approximate size of Salem-Keizer School District), you can expect around 120 new Level 1 meetings yearly. Approximately 55 percent will be elementary school students, 38 percent will be middle school students, and 7 percent will be high school students. Around half (65–75) of those Level 1 meetings will lead to a need for Level 2 consultation. Approximately 16 percent will be elementary school students, 20 percent will be middle school students, and 64 percent will be high school students. Around 60 percent of the cases identified through SIRC are SPED students.

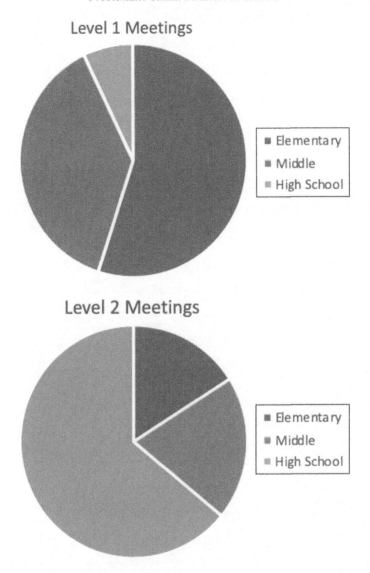

Level 1 Meetings

Legend:
- Elementary
- Middle
- High School

Level 2 Meetings

Legend:
- Elementary
- Middle
- High School

Take a look at those two pie charts. You'll notice that most of the Level 1 cases are in the elementary but that the overwhelming majority of those cases do not go to a Level 2. Conversely, you'll have comparatively fewer high school students who get identified for a Level 1, but the overwhelming majority of these cases go on to a Level 2. Although open to other interpretations, this data seems to indicate that most of the high school cases brought to a Level 1 are serious and likely to result in a Level 2, whereas the inverse is true for elementary students (i.e., these cases tend to be less serious and their supervision needs are easily addressed in a Level 1).

Chapter 3

On the Importance of Language

Okay! This is where our discussion of sexuality and sexual words begins. Before we get started, take a few deep breaths. The language you are about to encounter may be unfamiliar to you. Some of these words and these descriptions may make you feel embarrassed or foolish, but these words are very powerful and your mastery of them can be tremendously helpful to you. In the land of the easily embarrassed and sexually awkward, the person who can calmly and plainly say, "oral-genital contact" is king/queen.

The following is a list of sexual behaviors and sexual parts given in plain clinical language followed by some common colloquialisms (including all the colloquialisms would have doubled the length of this book). It is important that you use simple clinical language to talk about sexual behavior and sexual parts rather than colloquialisms because it signifies that you are a knowledgeable professional and it helps to create a feeling of safety for everyone in the room.

It is also important that you familiarize yourself with the list of common colloquialisms so that you can understand what less informed and possibly less educated people are talking about. Yes, some of the stuff on this list may seem pretty strange, but having this information will enable you to be prepared to intervene. Remember, it's not your goal to make judgments about these behaviors but to learn how to describe them in descriptive but non-offensive terms.

Clinical Language	Common Colloquialisms
Penis	pee-pee, dick, cock, johnson, junk, schlong, peter, thingy, privates
Testicles	balls, sack, nuts, nutsack, junk, nads
Vagina/vaginal area	yoo-hoo, vag, privates, hole, thingy, pussy, cunt, poon, poontang, twat, slit, bush, muff
Clitoris	clit, joy button, joy buzzer
Chest area	breasts, boobs, ta-tas, hooters, tits, titties
Frotteurism	dry humping, humping, leg humping
Sexual touching (self or with a partner)	masturbation, wanking, stroking off, jerking off, whacking off, spanking off, fingering, finger-banging, hand job, handy, hj, petting, old fashioned
Oral-genital contact	fellatio, cunnilingus, head, blow job, bj, hummer, go down on, suck off, eating out, top, throat
Oral-anal contact	analingus, rim job, tossed salad, eating out, eating ass
Vaginal penetration/ intercourse	sex, fucking, banging, humping, doing it, sleeping together, getting laid
Anal penetration	anal, butt sex, butt fucking, ass fucking, fudge packing
Forced/coerced sexual contact	rape
Voyeurism	peeping tom, peeper
Exhibitionism	disrobing in public, playing doctor, showing his penis/her vagina
Labia	pussy lips
Engaging in problematic sexual behavior	sexual offending
Orgasm	jizz, cum, spunk, squirt

You may notice that this list is far from complete and lacks many of the more unusual sexual behaviors or euphemisms. Generally, if you encounter an unusual word or phrase with which you are unfamiliar, consult the Internet (www.urbandictionary.com is a particularly useful site, but one that you will likely require special permission to access while at work). On the Internet you can find definitions for "rusty hook," "donkey punch," "Cincinnati Bundt cake," "Hot Carl," and a host of other unusual and shocking sexual behaviors to which you may hear students refer.

The other thing you will notice is that words like *sex, fellatio,* and *cunnilingus* ended up on the list of colloquialisms rather than the clinical language list. There is a reason for this. These words suggest a degree of mutual participation that should not be uniformly assumed. Again, it's vital to remember that sexual behavior, problematic or not, is BEHAVIOR first and foremost. All behavior is communication and all behavior can be understood and explained if the context is big enough. By letting go of fear and remaining curious, you will be better able to gather the important context that will help you understand, interpret, and explain the behavior.

Now, let's imagine you've just discovered two high school students engaged in "vaginal penetration" in the locker room. It is unwise to assume that these two students are having "sex," because the word "sex" suggests that the act was mutually agreed upon. It may be the case that one of the participants is not old enough to provide consent (which would suggest the possibility of statutory rape), or it may be the case that the "vaginal penetration" was not mutually agreed upon beforehand (which may suggest "forced/coerced sexual contact").

Regardless of all these possibilities, however, it can be mutually agreed upon that "vaginal penetration" occurred. If there are criminal charges to follow, that is law enforcement's responsibility to provide that language. Your job is simply to take what occurred and put it into simple clinical terms.

Allow me to provide an example of how to use simple clinical language taking the situation that occurred with Maggie's daughter, Coleen, and Janet.

Seth, the school administrator, holds a meeting in his office to further examine the situation that occurred between Coleen and Janet. In attendance are the school counselor, Janet's mother, Olivia, and a law enforcement officer.

Seth: "Thank you for coming to this meeting. I know it was short notice. The purpose of this meeting is to discuss Janet and make sure we are providing adequate support for her at school."

Olivia: "I think this is stupid . . . You're making a big deal out of a couple of girls playing doctor."

Seth: "Olivia, I understand your concern. I want you to know that the reason I think this meeting is so important is because I don't want things to get blown out of proportion. I don't really understand what has occurred but I want to make sure that we are doing everything we can to support Janet, and I'm really happy you are here. Maybe you could start by sharing what you know."

Olivia: "Most of what I know I learned from Maggie. The girls had a sleepover and the next day Coleen was saying Janet touched her yoo-hoo. I honestly don't know what happened. I tried to talk to Janet about it but she just clammed up. It's not a big deal though. All kids play doctor, right?"

Seth: "It's very common for children Janet's age to have an interest in their peers' bodies, but it is more unusual for them to engage in sexual touching. Right now, I'm not sure how concerned to be because I don't have much information. Let's start going over this protocol and we'll make a decision together about how concerning this behavior is once we get to the end of it. So, if I'm understanding you correctly, Coleen claims that Janet touched her vaginal area. Is that correct?"

Olivia: "Yes, that how I understand it."

By keeping the discussion focused, unemotional, and clinical, you help to set a professional tone that puts others as ease. Your role is to facilitate the gathering of information in a way that it is helpful and nonjudgmental, and you'll find that using clinical language helps to set the tone.

Take the parents' perspective for a moment. Hearing that your first-grade son gave oral sex to his peers in the restroom is much more devastating and terrifying than hearing that he engaged in oral-genital contact. The clinical language provides a degree of separation that helps parents turn down the emotion.

Conversely, clinical language also helps to express the seriousness of the situation. Oftentimes, especially with younger children, parents and administrators can easily minimize the seriousness of situation by using childlike terms to discuss serious sexual behavior. "David pulled down his pants and asked Billy to kiss his pee-pee," does not have the same resonance as, "David pulled down his pants and asked Billy to engage in oral genital contact." When you are initially walking into a problematic sexual situation, using clinical language is the key to finding that middle ground between overrepresenting the seriousness of a situation and minimizing it.

Instead of . . .	Use . . .
Had oral sex	Engaged in oral-genital contact
Put his fingers inside her vagina or anus	Digitally penetrated her vagina or anus
Had sex with	Vaginally penetrated or anally penetrated
Grabbed her boob	Touched her chest area
Masturbated in class	Touched herself sexually
Touched his pee-pee	Touched his penis

The most effective thing to do when developing this skill is to prepare your language in advance. Before meeting with parents, try to get a five-minute rundown from staff regarding the nature of the problematic sexual behavior, and write a few notes about the type of language you want to use for the conversation you're about to have. Being prepared in this way will enable you to handle even the toughest situations with professionalism.

OTHER TERMINOLOGY

Please remember to always avoid the terms "sexual offender" and "sexually offending" when discussing problematic sexual behavior. These terms are legal terms that belong to law enforcement and the judicial system. We have no business using them, and they will only serve to add tension and anxiety to your discussion (not to mention get you sued).

If there is evidence of sexual offending, we should always allow law enforcement or parole and probation officers to bring that language to the table. Further, you should strongly discourage all staff in your school from using this language to describe children with problematic sexual behavior.

For the purposes of the Level 2 process, the terms *problematic sexual behavior* or *sexually problematic behavior* simply refer to any remarkable and/or persistent sexual behavior that is being discouraged. This term can be used to describe any unwanted sexual behavior that staff and parents are attempting to inhibit. Even the lowly "peeing in the barkdust" can be considered "problematic sexual behavior" if it persists in spite of focused attempts to intervene.

While it is true that all SOs engage in problematic sexual behavior, and that most SOs evidenced problematic sexual behavior in their youth, it is not true that all those who evidence problematic sexual behavior will become SOs. In fact, research suggests that it is a very small percentage of adolescents who are identified as having problematic sexual behavior in their youth that go on to become sexual SOs as adults, regardless of whether they receive any treatment.

Although we may use this language in our Level 1 protocol, it is wise to discourage staff from referring to these students as "students with problematic sexual behavior." Schools are like little villages and although you may be doing your best to protect the FERPA (Family Educational Rights and Privacy Act) rights of the kids in your school, you have likely learned that interesting news easily spreads outside the school and into the community with remarkable speed. Parents volunteering in the classroom pick up that Suzie has been showing "problematic sexual behavior," or, God forbid, that Suzie is a "sex offender," and you can imagine that Suzie won't be getting many playdates after that news leaks into the coffee klatch.

Rather, it is important that when speaking to staff, you refer to these students as students with "boundary problems" and encourage them to do likewise. The term *boundary problems* can be used to describe children who will poke a peer in the eye when they stand too close, and it can be used to describe children who will attempt to touch peers sexually. It's a good, general term that lets staff and volunteering parents alike know that a child requires a higher degree of supervision without providing any specifics regarding the concerning behavior.

Describing these children as "children who have difficulty interacting with their peers," conveys the same message. It encourages supervisory staff and parents to be vigilant when observing the child, and to be on particular lookout for how these students interact with others.

Finally, a quick word about Gay/Lesbian/Bisexual/Transgendered/Queer/Intersex/Asexual/Allies and Others or GLBTQIA+ as this group is commonly referred. Please do not make the assumption that sexual behavior that occurs between members of the same sex is an indication of sexual or gender identity. Sometimes it is, sometimes it isn't, and you'll have no way of knowing.

Also, if you are working with a student who self-identifies as LGBTQIA+, please employ the same terminology and pronouns the student uses to describe him/her/themselves when referring to the student. Do not refer to these students as homosexual, as this is a term that is largely met with derision among members of LGBTQIA+ community. Further, when addressing transgendered youth, one should use the student's preferred pronouns.

Chapter 4

The Level 1 Protocol

The Level 1 protocol is a tool designed to help the Level 1 team determine how best to consider and address sexual behavior. It has three parts: Introduction, Survey, and Case Disposition. An example of a Level 1 protocol used by Salem-Keizer School District is included in appendix A. This protocol can be adapted to suit the needs of your district. For your edification, a visual flowchart of the Level 1 process is included in appendix C.

The agenda for the Level 1 meeting is as follows:

- Introduction
  ○ Inform team members of the purpose of the Level 1 meeting.
  ○ Detail the limitations of the Level 1 protocol.
- Survey Questions
- Case Disposition (Dismiss, Establish Supervision Plan, or Establish Supervision Plan, and Request a Level 2 Consultation)

If the case is not dismissed.

- Establish a Supervision Plan
- Set next meeting for review of Supervision Plan
- Request Level 2 Consultation if needed

INTRODUCTION

The Introduction states the purpose of the Level 1 meeting, establishes the limitations of the tool, and lays out the agenda for the Level 1 meeting.

The purpose of the Level 1 meeting is to determine if the sexual behavior in question is concerning or not, and how to address the behavior in the event that it is deemed to be of concern.

The limitations of this tool are as follows. The Level 1 protocol is not a risk assessment tool. It is not designed to provide actuarial risk information regarding the likelihood that an individual will engage in problematic sexual behavior in the future. The protocol is not an investigation tool. It is not designed to gather information that can be used to arrest or convict an individual. This protocol is also not a psychological evaluation tool. It doesn't reveal anything about the individual's intent, his or her mental state, personality, cognitive ability, or internal psychological processes.

Finally, the protocol is not a diagnostic tool. It does not diagnose sexual or psychological problems, and it should not be used as a mechanism for developing or ascribing diagnostic labels to an individual. It should be noted that any conclusions based upon this survey are time bound, and that the survey should be updated periodically to reflect the passage of time. Further, this survey should be updated as new and relevant information is gained about the problematic sexual behavior.

The Level 1 protocol is best thought of as a survey of the factors that are highly suggestive of concerning or problematic sexual behavior. It has only two purposes, to alert the Level 1 team that they need additional consultation and to help them develop a supervision plan. Although this tool is not intended to be used for forensic application, it is important that all team members understand that, like any part of a student's school record, the information gathered in this tool is subject to subpoena.

LEVEL 1 SURVEY QUESTIONS

Now that we've got the meeting underway, we can examine the Level 1 Survey Questions. The Level 1 Survey Questions gather information in a number of areas that research suggests may be indicative of a concerning or problematic sexual behavior. Remember, the term *concerning or problematic sexual behavior* refers to any sexual behavior that is unwanted and/or continues in spite of intervention.

Sometimes you will have a situation where the child's parent is unable to attend the Level 1 team meeting or where a teacher has valuable information but cannot attend the Level 1. In the event of such a situation, you may want to use a semi-structured interview as a means of gathering useful information. You will find examples of semi-structured interviews of this sort in appendix B. Please note that the questions in these tools correspond to the Level 1 protocol. Specifically, the numbers in parentheses after each question correspond to the relevant questions on the Level 1 protocol.

The following is a list of questions you are encouraged to include in your Level 1 Survey as well as the rationale for including that question. Please bear in mind that the answers to these questions are important not only because they help you understand how serious the behavior is, but also because they provide you useful information that will be necessary for developing a supervision/intervention plan.

1. Are the individuals involved in the sexual incident roughly equivalent with regard to age, development, cognitive capacity, physical capacity, emotional functioning, and coping skills?

Sexual incidents that occur between children, who are not roughly equivalent with regard to development, may reflect a power imbalance. It is important to consider not only differences in age, but also differences in physical size and capacity, intelligence, and emotional capacity, because differences in these areas can make individuals more vulnerable.

For example, there can be a tremendous difference in the physical size between two thirteen-year-old males. Thought of in the context of sexual misbehavior, one can imagine that physical size gives a person an advantage that cannot be accounted for by age alone. The same is true for intelligence, or emotional capacity.

It's not uncommon in this era of mainstreaming, that kids with varying cognitive abilities share the same classroom. Imagine the following scenario: a sixteen-year-old male of normal cognitive ability makes a habit of romantically pursuing cognitively delayed same-aged female peers. Technically, these individuals are same-aged and so this behavior would not be easily adjudicated. However, there is little doubt that this boy's sexual behavior is targeted, intentional, and harmful.

It's important to keep this in mind with your emotionally vulnerable populations as well. Children who qualify under Emotional Behavioral Disability, Autism Spectrum Disorder, or who otherwise evidence psychological problems, can be more easily preyed upon by others sexually. Consequently, we have a greater responsibility to protect these students and to carefully scrutinize their romantic relationships to prevent victimization. This is not to imply that one make a habit of routinely interfering in these relationships. Rather, this suggests that we need to be on the lookout for individuals who are consistently targeting our more vulnerable populations.

So how big of a difference in development, or size or cognitive capacity is worth noting? Generally, it's wise to look to the laws in your state for guidance. In most states, a difference of more than three years in age is grounds for criminal consideration. So, generally, looking for physical, developmental, cognitive and/or emotional differences that are suggestive of a three-year gap seems like a wise approach.

2. Is there a known history of previous sexually inappropriate behavior?

This one is kind of a no-brainer. If you have a student with a history of problematic sexual behavior, it is more likely that the sexual behavior that caused you to initiate a Level 1 is of concern. Remember, the best predictor of future behavior for kids with sexual misbehavior is past behavior. If the student evidences a history of sexual misbehavior, it's more likely that you will need a higher level of supervision and intervention, and that you may need to seek consultation.

3. Has this student been previously censured, disciplined, or placed on a behavior/safety plan for sexually inappropriate behavior?

Again, another obvious one, right? You don't need a PhD to understand that a student who has been placed on a supervision plan for sexual misbehavior is probably a student who struggles with problematic sexual behavior. If that student violated the supervision plan in a sexual way, you should be even more concerned. Any problematic sexual behavior that continues in spite of intervention is very serious and in need of immediate attention and significant intervention.

4. Has the student been exposed to inappropriate sexual content or behavior?

Kids who have been prematurely exposed to inappropriate sexual content or behavior often evidence problematic sexualized behavior in response to this exposure. Consequently, if you have evidence that a child has seen pornography, been exposed to adult sexual behavior, or been the victim of sexual assault, it is important to note that these factors may be important to consider when thinking about the seriousness of the behavior, and with regard to safety planning.

5. Is there consensus among the parties involved in the sexual incident regarding what occurred?

Oftentimes, the parties involved in a sexual incident disagree about what occurred. This disagreement can be the result of several factors. Disagreement could suggest confusion about the incident, poor communication skills, differences in perspective or some other element. In some cases, disagreement also reflects the possibility that one or more parties to the sexual incident are intentionally being deceptive.

Whatever the reason, disagreement about the facts should alert you that there are additional complexities to the situation that must be considered. Where are the stories consistent and where do they diverge? Does one party appear to have the upper hand in the incident? What reasons might there be for the inconsistency in the stories? It's not your job to determine what actually happened, but it is your task as a team to give serious consideration to the information you have in front of you, and do your utmost to make sense out of it.

6. Were coercive or manipulative measures used to get compliance with the sexual incident or encourage secrecy?

In other words, did one or more of the parties to the incident use threats or otherwise attempt to manipulate others into participating in the sexual incident or keeping the incident a secret. The use of coercion or manipulation suggests that undue pressure was used to gain compliance.

Clearly, individuals who put undue pressure on others sexually are not engaged in normative, developmentally appropriate sexual behavior. Rather, this sort of sexual behavior is potentially more harmful and concerning because it suggests that consent or assent was not freely given. Additionally, individuals who employ this method to gain sexual compliance generally evidence less regard for how their sexual behavior impacts others.

One must also give serious consideration to how much effort was made to maintain secrecy about the sexual behavior. Individuals who put undue pressure on others to maintain secrecy about sexual behavior are generally aware that the behavior is considered inappropriate and are attempting to avoid the consequences of that sexual behavior being discovered.

It is important to understand that coercion and manipulation can take many forms. Gift giving, granting privileges, and favoritism can be just as compelling as threatening to harm someone when you are attempting to keep something hidden.

7. Was the sexual behavior developmentally normative?

Developmentally normative sexual behavior in children is an area in which very little research has been conducted, probably because this is a domain that most adults would like to pretend doesn't exist. Adults don't like to think about children as sexual beings. It squicks us out. But if you think back to your own childhood, you will recall funny feelings, strange sensations, and curiosity about your "private parts" that occurred well before you hit puberty. Wondering what is going on "down there" is all very normal, even in very young children.

So how do we tell what is normal and what is not?

First, we will address prepubescent children. If a young child is evidencing unusual interest in their genitals all of a sudden, it's always wise to start by looking for a medical cause. Sometimes what appears to be sexual rubbing or preoccupation with one's genitals can be explained by a simple infection or an easily remedied medical problem. Remember to pay close attention, however, to recurrent medical problems in the genital area as this can sometimes be suggestive of neglect, poor medical care, or, in some cases, sexual victimization.

Generally speaking, it is unusual for prepubescent children to have much knowledge about or interest in penetrative or adult sexual behavior.

They shouldn't naturally have much interest in sex until their bodies get flooded with the sex hormones that accompany puberty. Most prepubescent kids consider adult sexual behavior yucky. The most typical response to a description of adult sexual behavior should be "ewwww!"

Most kids under the age of around thirteen or so may be a little curious about "privates." They may be okay with looking at their peers' genitals or showing off their own in private, but the thought of genital contact is usually considered gross. When they do engage in "playing doctor," the play is typically lighthearted and silly, not goal directed or pressured, and it is unusual for any genital contact to occur. Although this sort of sexual play is considered normal, that is not to suggest that you encourage it. A simple message like, "exploring your body is okay, but it's something you do on your own, in private," should suffice.

This is not true of children who have been prematurely exposed to adult sexual behavior. These children may express knowledge and interest about adult sexual behavior that is not easily curbed by a simple talking to. They understand the basic mechanics of sex and may seek out genital contact and adult sexual behavior with other children or adults. Their sexual behavior with others is typically goal directed and focused. These kids may make sexual sounds and gestures and they may appear sexualized or flirtatious.

It's not uncommon for adults to see this type of problematic sexualized behavior in children and jump to the conclusion that these children have been sexually victimized. While it is always the case that there is an underlying cause for the problematic sexualized behavior, *do not make the mistake of thinking that children who have been prematurely exposed to adult sexual behavior have been sexually molested.*

Oftentimes there is a concerning, but much more banal explanation. Sometimes it's as simple as "Johnny has a sixteen-year-old brother who is sexually active and who talks openly about it in front of him." In other cases, the culprit might be exposure to pornography, loose sexual boundaries around the house, or sexually promiscuous parents who are not doing a good job protecting their children from their sexual exploits. The aforementioned situations are potentially harmful to children, they may warrant reporting to law enforcement, and they can lead to problematic sexual behavior, but they fall far short of sexual molestation.

Okay, on to adolescents. Although we hate to think about it and we sure don't condone it, it's not considered pathological for adolescent kids to have knowledge about and interest in penetrative and adult sexual behavior. Kids in the thirteen and older age range generally view adult sexual behavior as interesting and potentially sexually arousing. They are no longer grossed out by the thought of sex (although they likely still find it appalling to talk to adults about it), and they are starting to think about it more and starting to actively pursue it with peers.

Because adolescents tend to sexually function more like adults, it can seem tricky to determine when things are developmentally off track. The key here is to look at features of the sexual encounter that suggest an unhealthy process is at play. Sexual contact with nonpeers, coercive or forceful sexual contact, public sexual behavior or paraphilic (i.e., markedly atypical or unusual sexual behavior) behavior suggests there may be a larger problem.

We've spent some time on the importance of considering developmental factors regarding sexual contact between peers, and we've discussed the concern about coercive sexual contact, but we haven't said much about public sexual behavior or paraphilic interest. Sometimes the location of a sexual behavior, rather than the act itself, is the primary concern. The schoolyard, an abandoned school office, a porta-potty, a public restroom, the locker room, or the back of the bus are not places for sex. If students are caught engaging in sexual behavior in these areas, regardless of whether or not it's peer-to-peer or consensual, it should be considered noteworthy and examined more closely. While it's possible that nothing untoward was occurring, it's worth digging a little more deeply.

Paraphilia literally means "other love." It is a term used to describe sexual interests and behavior that fall outside of what is generally considered the norm. In the common vernacular, paraphilic behavior is often referred to as "kink," and includes things like sadomasochistic behavior, bondage and discipline, fetish (sexual interest in objects), partialism (sexual interest in specific body parts, e.g., feet), pedophilia, voyeurism, exhibitionism, zoophilia, and a host of other less typical sexual behaviors too numerous to easily list.

Although many paraphilic behaviors, such as sadomasochism, cross-dressing, fetish, and partialism (sexual preoccupation with body parts), are generally believed to be non-problematic as long as they are engaged in with a consenting peer, some paraphilic behaviors (pedophilia, zoophilia, necrophilia) are considered deviant, problematic, and potentially harmful to others. Consequently, it's important to pay close attention to situations that are suggestive of paraphilic behavior, especially if it occurs in the thirteen and under crowd. Please note: LGBTQIA+ behaviors are not considered fundamentally deviant or paraphilic so you are going to need to look at what sexual behavior is occurring and how it is occurring rather than pathologizing sexual behavior based solely upon the genders of those involved.

So, a quick review of developmentally unusual sexual behavior; in kids around the age of thirteen and under, any behavior that suggests knowledge about or interest in adult sexual behavior should be considered unusual. In kids around the age of thirteen and older, any sexual behavior that is coercive, not peer-to-peer, paraphilic or occurs in a public space should be considered unusual. And lastly, just because a child evidences unusual or problematic sexual behavior does not mean he or she has been molested. Rather, it suggests some premature exposure to adult sexual behavior.

8. Was anyone physically or emotionally harmed as a result of the sexual incident?

Another easy one. Any sexual situation in which one of the individuals identifies as or appears as having been victimized warrants further scrutiny. Let me be clear. It's not your job to determine if someone was actually victimized or to mete out justice. That is the role of law enforcement. It's your job, as a Level 1 team, to consider this information when you are deciding if you need additional consultation, and when you are developing a supervision plan.

Victimization suggests that the situation was unwanted or was in some way upsetting. It could suggest that one of the individuals in the sexual situation was callous or unconcerned about the well-being of others; it could suggest that there was confusion or poor communication about the sexual situation, or it could be suggestive of other complex processes. You don't need to get to the bottom of it, and you can always pass it along to the Level 2 consultation team (that we'll talk about in the next chapter) if you are confused about the implications of the victimization. Just don't ignore it if you have evidence.

9. How does the student explain the sexual behavior? Was there confusion about the appropriateness of the sexual behavior?

Sometimes you will run across problematic sexual behaviors in children that are the result of confusion about the appropriateness of specific sexual behavior. Some children grow up in environments where sexual behavior and sexual talk are commonplace.

As crazy as it sounds, these sorts of kids simply don't get that their behavior is unusual because sexual behavior is a routine part of their daily experience. They may have parents who watch pornography in front of them on a regular basis, or who have no reservations about engaging in sexual behavior in front of their children. As a result, these kids are socialized to engage in adult sexual behavior at a young age, and it doesn't seem odd to them.

Differing cultural norms and challenges with acculturation can also account for confusion about the appropriateness of sexual behavior. Many cultures are much less reserved about physical touching than what is commonly experienced in mainstream America.

This is not to suggest that the behavior be ignored on the basis of cultural differences. It is obviously very important to encourage children to engage in socially acceptable behavior. However, it is also important to consider the possibility that an unusual sexual behavior might be a reflection of confusion over a cultural norm rather than a sign of sexual deviance.

Children with severe cognitive deficits (below fifty IQ) may also have difficulty understanding that a specific sexual behavior is inappropriate and they may evidence considerable confusion about why they shouldn't engage in a certain behavior that simply feels so good. For many of these severely impaired kids, the sexually gratifying behavior in which they are engaging has no real connection to sexuality in the sense we think about it.

To many kids with severe cognitive impairments, it's not a sex act in the conventional sense but just a thing they do that feels great, like scratching an itch. They don't get why it creeps everyone out. Be mindful though, regardless of the underlying cause, you still need to put a plan in place to decrease the behavior and protect others. Simply put, regardless of intent, the behaviors themselves are problematic and need to be addressed.

It is also worth noting that just because a child has low IQ doesn't mean they can't have more devious motives underlying their sexual behavior. There are plenty of individuals with low IQ who are remarkably interpersonally savvy and who are also predatory, pedophilic, or criminally minded with regard to their problematic sexual behavior. So be mindful that IQ tests don't do great job of evaluating all aspects of intelligence.

10. Is there an imbalance of power between the individuals involved in the sexual incident?

An imbalance of power (remarkable differences in size, physical strength, emotional stability, access to opportunity/resources, and social standing) can be used to encourage or coerce others into sexual behavior. The power differential can often be very subtle and it doesn't need to be obviously stated in order to work. Individuals who depend upon a power differential for sexual gratification often target vulnerable individuals for sexual behavior because they are more compliant and less likely to reveal victimization.

11. Was a weapon present during the sexual incident?

The mere presence of a weapon during sexual behavior, regardless of whether it was used in a threatening way or even made reference to, may suggest that coercion was employed. It should be noted that the term *weapon* refers to any object that may be used to threaten physical or emotional safety and is not limited to conventional weapons such as knives or firearms.

12. Was grooming behavior employed leading up to the sexual incident?

Grooming behavior is a fancy sex offender term that is often used to describe the behaviors that pedophiles or predatory SOs employ to gain victims' trust as they work toward permeating their physical boundaries for the purpose of sexually molesting them. In truth, grooming behavior is not any different from flirtatious behavior in how it presents. It's the same sort of behavior you engaged in when attempting to pick up a sexual partner in your wilder days. You look longingly into her eyes. You casually touch his hand or rub your foot against his. You talk sweetly and lovingly. You give gifts (or buy dinner). You talk about the special connection you feel for one another.

There is nothing wrong with this type of behavior when it occurs among mutually interested, developmentally similar peers around the age of thirteen and older. However, grooming behavior should be very carefully considered when it is evidenced in prepubescent kids (remember they shouldn't have much interest in sex or flirtatious behavior before puberty) or when a child uses it with a less developmentally competent (younger) youth as it suggests a familiarity with adult sexual behavior, targeting, and potential manipulativeness.

13. Does the sexual incident give you a strong visceral response (i.e., make you feel uneasy)?

People generally find this last question to be a bit odd as a part of the protocol, but there is good clinical evidence that your gut reaction is a worthwhile investigative tool. It's not the only one you should use, mind you, but it is important.

Sometimes, that old reptilian, fight-or-flight part of the brain kicks in for reasons that we can't readily explain. You'll encounter situations where things just don't add up, or you are left feeling uneasy without any one thing you can pin that feeling on. It would be absolutely nuts to make an important decision about a child's life based upon that feeling, but it would be completely rational to request additional consultation. That's why this question is so important. It's the one that allows you to sleep well at night because you didn't have to make the tough call on a situation that just didn't feel right.

14. Other Concerns

Frequently, there are a host of complicating concerns that are not specific to the problematic sexual behavior but that should be considered because they impact your intervention strategies. Does this child have a history of harmful behavior toward animals? Is there any current suicidal ideation? Has she made targeted threats of violence? Has he struggled with enuresis (bedwetting) or encopresis (soiling themselves)?

Is there a history of harming animals? Is there DHS/foster care involvement? Are there complicating mental health concerns? Physical health concerns? Relevant historical factors (significant life events, serious losses, trauma)? Has the student been exposed to physical or sexual abuse, neglect or domestic violence? Familial incarceration?

How's the kid's current mental state (any big changes in sleep, mood, appetite, activity level or school performance)? Gathering information about these domains helps you get a handle on potential areas where intervention might be needed and it gives you a sense for resources that are already being utilized.

CASE DISPOSITION

Once you have completed the section on Other Concerns, the Level 1 team must make a decision regarding the disposition of the case. You have three options.

1. Dismiss the case as unconcerning.
2. Develop a Supervision and Intervention Plan which you will review periodically to determine if it is effective.
3. Develop a Supervision and Intervention Plan which you will review periodically to determine if it is effective *and* request Level 2 Consultation.

So, how do you make the decision? You should strive to come to a consensus via discussion of the survey questions. In the event that consensus is not possible (which is unusual), however, the administrator should be the final decision maker because she or he is ultimately responsible for the security and safety of the school.

It's not very hard to tell when a case is unconcerning. Everyone looks at the information and agrees that the potential harm to others and seriousness of the behavior is negligible. Any other decision, however, warrants a supervision plan (you'll get a chapter on that next).

If the team agrees that the behavior can be sufficiently addressed by the school via supervision and intervention strategies, then a supervision/intervention plan is developed and put into action, and a date is set to review the efficacy of that plan. Should the team decide, however, to seek consultation from the Level 2 consultation team, then a temporary supervision/intervention plan should be put into action immediately while the school-based Level 1 team is awaiting feedback from the multiagency Level 2 consultation team.

Chapter 5

Addressing Resistance

Sexually problematic behavior is absolutely terrifying to most people. Some people will stand out in the rain for days to protest the execution of murderers, but even the most liberal-minded folks have very little regard for the welfare of sex offenders. Sex offenders are, without question, considered by many to be among the lowest of the low, and the vilest degenerates of society.

In truth, the overwhelming majority of individuals who commit sexual crimes are just incredibly damaged human beings who are capable of change, but saying that doesn't alter how society views them. That being said, when you are meeting with parents to discuss their child's concerning sexual behavior, or talking about this issue with staff, everyone's biggest fear is that you are telling them this child is a sex offender.

Given that context, resistance is normal and should be expected. That bears repeating, resistance is normal and should be expected. If anything, be concerned if the parent or guardian seems unconcerned or overly punitive toward the student. Although it's impossible to anticipate every way in which parents or other staff might react, this chapter provides you some strategies for addressing common forms of resistance.

RESISTANCE AS A RESULT OF CONCERN OVER FACTS

Oftentimes, when parents or staff are confronted with children's concerning sexual behavior that they didn't witness, their first instinct is to protect their child by getting into an argument over "what really happened." You may hear people saying things like, "How can you know for certain if no one saw it?" and, "It's he said/she said."

Because you'll never know the facts of what really occurred, it's very easy to lose focus by getting into a pointless discussion in an attempt to establish the facts. Remember that establishing the facts is the responsibility of law enforcement. Let's take a look at how Seth handles this very common argument regarding confusion about the facts.

Olivia (Janet's mom): "Look. Coleen is a liar. I've never been able to trust that kid. And I'm not going to sit here and put my daughter on the hot seat just because Coleen is making up stories. We don't know what happened, and we'll never know what happened. You can't even prove anything. This is a waste of time and I won't have my daughter punished for something you can't even prove."

Seth: "Olivia, I understand your concern. And I'm equally frustrated by the situation. I really wish we knew for certain what, if anything, happened between Janet and Coleen. You're correct. It's information that is beyond our grasp. But this isn't a criminal investigation and we're not here to establish the facts or punish anyone."

"Allow me to explain my concern and why I think we need to have this meeting. Regardless of what actually occurred, we have some concerning allegations in front of us. My goal for this meeting today is not that we make a determination about the facts and dole out punishment, but that we work together to create a plan so that these sorts of allegations do not arise again. It is very important to me that we protect Janet's reputation in the school and in the community and I think we can do that by developing a solid supervision plan."

You are not a criminal investigator. It is not your job to get every detail. You don't need to determine exactly what happened. You are not the finder of facts. It's not your job to get to the bottom of things, and it's important that everyone understand that.

It is, however, your job to create a safe school environment. You can accomplish this by carefully considering any allegations of concerning behavior and addressing them in a consistent manner. In so doing, you protect the students and staff in your school and you protect the reputations of your students who may be exhibiting problematic sexual behavior. By shifting the discussion from an unsolvable problem (not knowing the facts) to a concrete solution (protecting the reputation of students), you can help to move the discussion forward and set parents' minds at ease.

PASSIVE RESISTANCE

Sometimes parents and/or staff respond to allegations of concerning behavior in children with what is best described as passive resistance. These individuals may recognize that there is some problematic sexual behavior but they either won't or can't do the things they need to address the behavior. Sometimes these folks are simply too overwhelmed with the daily difficulties of life to effectively address the problematic sexual behavior.

In some cases, these people just don't see the sexual behavior as a problem, or they view the supervision plan as punitive, and so they give lip service to what the administrator is asking them to do while not actually making any attempts to solve the problem. Occasionally, you may have the misfortune of running into a person who reacts with passive resistance to any form of authority or control.

Passive resistance is best met with a frank discussion regarding the nature of liability, followed by an offer of support. In attempting to address the situation between John and Raymond, Liz puts a supervision plan in place at school that involves keeping these two away from one another, but Liz just got an angry call from Raymond's father that John has been bullying Raymond again at school and that the classroom teacher, Karl has been largely ignoring the supervision plan for weeks.

Liz: "Karl, I just got a call from Raymond's dad. He said that John has been bullying Raymond for the last two weeks. I was under the impression that they weren't allowed to play together anymore as per the supervision plan."

Karl: "I don't think it's a big deal, Liz. We don't really know what happened with those boys, if anything. I try to keep them apart, but you know how busy I am. It's just not that important."

Liz: "You're right, Karl. We don't know what happened with those boys. We don't know if John instigated something, or if Raymond was the instigator. And I do know how busy you are, believe me. But here's my concern. Regardless of what did or didn't happen, we now have to consider our liability for future incidents. If something happens in the future between these boys, we will appear negligent if we didn't do our utmost to prevent it.

My concern is that you will be considered liable because you didn't follow the supervision plan we outlined, and I want to protect you from that. You are a valuable teacher and I want to make sure I don't lose you. So please, let me know how I can be helpful to you in making sure the plan gets followed."

Karl: "I guess I wasn't really thinking of it like that. But you're right. I don't want to be the weak link here. I think I'm having the hardest time providing supervision to them during recess. Do you have any ideas about how I could do that?"

Liz could just as easily have used this approach with a parent who was passively resistant to following the supervision plan. The argument is essentially the same. Once allegations of problematic sexual behavior have been communicated, every person (parents, staff, administrators, community stakeholders) who heard those allegations bears some liability.

Failure to follow through with protective measures can lead to serious consequences and carry legal ramifications. It's important that everyone at the table, everyone who is responsible for carrying out a supervision plan, understand the weight of their role and how to get the help they need in order to adequately address their own liability.

HOSTILE RESISTANCE

In many situations, the resistance we are met with is far more obvious, direct and hostile. It's not uncommon to run into people who address difficulties with a "scorched earth" policy, and they aren't difficult to identify. This is the person screaming profanity at you on the phone, this is the person threatening to "lawyer up" if you don't give in, this is the person pulling their child out of your school unless you make the supervision plan go away, and this is the person who doesn't show up to the Level 1 meeting. They are as subtle as a train wreck in their tactics.

In dealing with hostile resistance keep one notion in mind, "you cannot negotiate with terrorists." There is no discussion with someone who is using abusive language. This may mean hanging up on a verbally abusive phone call, or calling an end to a meeting if people are not using respectful language.

Should a party decide to lawyer up, remind them that you need to know when they are bringing their attorney so that you can have the school's attorney present at those meetings as well. If parents attempt to move their child to a different school or a different district or pull their child out of school completely, make sure that the important safety concerns (and the liability) you have, get handed off to the appropriate decision makers.

Finally, in the event that a party doesn't show up to the Level 1 meeting, have that meeting without them. Safety and supervision are of the utmost importance and should not be waylaid by stalling tactics.

OVERCOMPLIANCE

One must also be on the lookout for the opposite of resistance: overcompliance. Consider what occurs when Kelly, our high school counselor finally meets with Brian's mother, Mary, to discuss Brian's behavior.

Kelly: "Hi, I'm Brian's school counselor. As I spoke to you about on the phone, Brian has been evidencing some problematic sexual behavior at school. Today we're going to be going over a Level 1 Protocol that will help us learn a little more about Brian's problematic sexual behavior and we'll consider how he might be helped by a supervision plan. Do you have any questions before we get started?"

Mary: "I don't got any questions. But I sure can tell you a lot about that little pervert. He's been doing this kinda crap for years. Even got into trouble a while back for diddling his little sister. I've been trying to get the school to set him straight for forever, but they don't do nothing. He's the kinda little creep doesn't learn to keep his hand outta the cookie jar unless it gets slapped enough."

Clearly, Mary sees a possibility that she can use the school as a punitive instrument and is hopeful that the Level 1 process will be some form of punishment. It's important that everyone understand that the Level 1 protocol and the resulting supervision plan are not punishment or in any way linked to your school disciplinary system. Although supervision plans often place limitations on the behaviors of students for the purpose of increasing safety, they are not intended to be, and should not be, used punitively.

Again, keep in mind that resistance is to be expected, and that, in some ways, lack of resistance may be an indicator that there is a problem. Resistance, on its own, doesn't indicate that a person has bad intentions. Typically, it communicates protectiveness, which is a good thing. We are more likely, however, to get compliance when we can help parents and staff realize that they can be most protective to the student by engaging in the Level 1 process and by following the supervision plan.

Chapter 6

Supervision/Intervention

The traditional model for threat assessment suggests that there are three overlapping factors that need to be considered when mitigating threat: intent, opportunity, and access. Thought of within the context of suicide, violence, or fire setting, this model holds together well. In order to commit suicide, set a fire, or harm others, you need to have the intent to cause harm, access to a tool for creating harm (weapon, overdose pills, matches, and so on), and the opportunity to harm. Unfortunately, this model doesn't work as well with regard to problematic sexual behavior.

Without question, the easiest of these three factors to control is access. Limit a person's access to lethal means and you've seriously impacted the harm they can do to themselves or others. A firebug can't wreak much harm at your school if you search him every day for combustible material. The problem with applying this model to problematic sexual behavior is it's very difficult to determine exactly what the "tool for creating harm" is and how to limit access to it.

Before a potential school shooter is able to act on his intent he reaches for a gun, before a firebug can act on his intent he reaches for the matches. But what does an individual with problematic sexual behavior reach for? What is their destructive tool? Is it their hand? Their genitals? Their mind? Pornography? It's hard to say. And even if you could say for certain, how can you limit access? We can't remove these "tools for creating harm" or limit access to them except via the most archaic means.

Instead of attempting to get this three-factor model to fit when it doesn't, and wasting our time trying to figure out what is meant by access, it's better to just consider the two factors that you can assess and hopefully impact: intent and opportunity.

Let's look briefly at intent. Intent is the desire to act, in this case, in a sexually harmful manner. It may be the desire to sexually molest, rape, sexually harass, sexually intimidate, groom or sexually satisfy oneself in some way that causes harm or discomfort (such as public masturbation or frotteurism). Intent is the thought that leads to the action. Individuals with low or no intent to harm others sexually are much less likely to engage in sexually harmful behavior than those who have a strong intent to harm others sexually.

There is some good news and some bad news about intent. The bad news is this: research has repeatedly demonstrated that sexual desire (intent) is incredibly difficult to change. The good news is that it is not the job of schools to try and change intent.

The difficult job of impacting intent belongs to mental health professionals. Your job is simply to help individuals with problematic sexual behavior get access to mental health professionals in your area who can help them with their problematic sexual intent. Once you have made this hand off, the tough work of changing intent belongs to the mental health professionals and the person being treated.

Having just orchestrated this successful hand off to the mental health professionals in your area, you can now set your mind to the far easier task of addressing opportunity. Opportunity refers to the where, when, and how of problematic sexual behavior. Where do you think it is most likely to occur? What times of the day or in which situations is there the greatest risk? How is the problematic sexual behavior likely to manifest? Let's consider an example.

Amanda is a nine-year-old female in third grade. She engages in a lot of sexual talk at school and in the community, and seems to have very unusual boundaries around adult men. Amanda will attempt to hug and sit on the lap of any adult male she meets, and her demeanor toward adult males is overtly flirtatious.

Amanda has been repeatedly reprimanded over the last three years for touching her peers inappropriately during recess, floor time, and when standing in line. Recently she was caught in the girl's room attempting to digitally penetrate the vagina of a first-grade girl who was attempting to use the restroom.

Imagine you are reviewing a Level 1 protocol on Amanda. Is the other child involved in the incident her developmental equivalent? No. Does she have a history of sexually inappropriate behavior? Yes. Has she been censured for her sexual behavior in the past? Yes. Is this behavior developmentally normative? No. Did the other child feel victimized? Was manipulation used? Did grooming occur?

Your questioning around the incident will enable you to answer these others questions. But even on the basis of the first few questions and the description of the event, there is very little question that this is a child who (1) needs help with her problematic sexual behavior, (2) should be referred to a Level 2 Team, and (3) requires a supervision plan.

You already know how to refer Amanda to the Level 2 Team, and you know how to get her help with her problematic sexual behavior (refer her and her family to a qualified mental health professional). Your task now is protecting your school and the community. You've already got the most important people in Amanda's life in the room (since you just completed the Level 1), so now is the perfect time to switch the focus to intervention and supervision.

A quick thing about supervision—No child likes being on supervision. They often complain and try to find reasons to avoid this at any cost. Parents generally feel the same way. They fear their children will be ostracized or made to stand out because they are being supervised. So, before you start to move forward with a supervision plan, it is usually important to help everyone at the table understand what the purpose is.

Supervision planning should accomplish several tasks.

- Ensure the safety of others
- Protect the reputation of the student in need of supervision
- Clearly delineate who holds liability in which situations
- Improve accountability by clearly outlining tasks and assigning responsibilities to student, staff, and parents for keeping the school and community safe
- Articulate a process for handling unexpected situations
- Make clear what conditions need to exist before supervision can be reduced

Let's look at each of these points in a little more detail.

Obviously, the most important reason to implement a supervision/intervention plan is to protect others. It's important when developing these plans that one remember that protection doesn't just cover students but also staff at the school and others in the community. A good supervision plan will keep the kids in your school safe, but it will also protect your staff from sexual assault as well as from false allegations from sexually reactive students. Further, your plan should also include strategies to protect the community at large, including church groups, afterschool activities, community centers, and others venues. We'll talk more about how to do that later in this chapter.

The importance of protecting the reputation of the student with problematic sexual behavior really can't be emphasized enough. Most parents react very strongly to having their child on a supervision plan for problematic sexual behavior. They fear their child will be labeled a pervert and consequently ostracized by society, but a good supervision/intervention plan can help prevent that by making sure that sensitive information about a student is well protected, and by limiting the likelihood that the child will engage in future harmful sexual behavior.

A good supervision plan makes it clear who holds the liability in which situations. It eliminates the "I didn't know it was my responsibility" phenomenon by making it known to parents, school staff, and community partners whose job it is to provide supervision in which situations. Further, a good supervision plan formally documents the agreement that parents, school staff, and community partners are entering into toward the goal of improving safety. Should a second problematic sexual incident arise after establishing a safety plan, it will be patently clear who dropped the ball and where the responsibility lies.

It is impossible to have any accountability or control liability without the assignment of supervision tasks. A good supervision plan makes it known to everyone what their roles are in which situations toward the improvement of safety. Further, it documents these roles and clarifies these responsibilities in such a way that it makes these roles easy to follow and clearly delineated.

Because one cannot reasonably account for every possibility, it's important that good supervision plans include plans for how to addresses failures or lapses in supervision. What if there is a substitute teacher? How will you handle it if your school resource officer is out on maternity leave? What if the student is dropped off late to school? A good supervision plan includes potential "what if" scenarios and makes it known what to do when things don't go according to the plan.

Finally, a good supervision plan makes it clear what conditions need to be met prior to reducing the level of supervision. We'll get to more on that later.

EXAMINING THE DAY

As we go through the following sections, it might be helpful to have a copy of the supervision portion of the Level 1 protocol in front of you. You can find it on pages ten and eleven of the Level 1 protocol in appendix A.

Always begin every supervision meeting with a detailed discussion of the student's day. How does the student get to school? Is there a need for supervision during transport between school and home? Clearly, any student who is sexually harming others while on the bus, while walking to school, or while walking to and from the bus, needs supervision in these environments.

How you choose to address the concern is up to you and the Level 1 Team. You may decide that the student needs an assigned seat on the bus, close to supervision, or that the student needs supervision while walking to school, or while walking to and from the bus. The manner in which you address the concern should (1) align with district policy and procedures, (2) fit the supervision needs of the student, and (3) make clear the roles of important adult supervisors.

"Amanda had three incidents of touching other students on the bus last year, so if she is going to continue to ride the bus, she needs to be in a seat by herself directly to the right of the bus driver, or she could be driven to school by her parents."

When the student gets to school, should she be allowed to immediately comingle with her peers or does she need to wait in a designated supervised area until class starts? If she needs supervision, where will it occur and who will be responsible for it?

"Based on her history it appears that Amanda takes advantage of less structured times to touch others sexually. We could have her wait in the office with the secretaries until her teacher can escort her to class, or we could have her go to the gym where several other kids meet in the morning. Ms. Ingvaldsen supervises the gym in the morning, so as long as we tell her to keep an eye on Amanda, that should work fine. I'd rather have Amanda in the gym so that she can socialize, but let's keep the office idea in mind in case Amanda is too hard to manage in the gym."

LINE-OF-SIGHT SUPERVISION

Once at school, will the child require "line-of-sight" supervision or "arm's-reach" supervision? Any student on a supervision plan is technically "line-of-sight," meaning that they must always be in "line-of-sight" of a "knowledgeable adult supervisor." Let's talk about "line-of-sight" first, and we'll get to "arm's-reach" and "knowledgeable adult supervisor" in a minute.

Any student with an unresolved history of problematic sexual behavior should be on "line-of-sight" supervision. This may seem difficult to provide, especially in our era of huge financial cutbacks, where resources are limited, but in fact, you are probably providing darn near "line-of-sight" supervision to every kid in your school.

All of your students receive "line-of-sight" supervision in the classroom, in the cafeteria, and while on recess. The real gaps in "line-of-sight" are likely occurring during passing periods or when a student is going to use the restroom. So, when you a put a "line-of-sight" supervision plan in place, you really need to focus on two things, making sure your "knowledgeable adult supervisors" know what they need to do, and filling in these little gaps in "line-of-sight."

PASSING PERIODS, RECESS, BATHROOMS, AND CAFETERIA SUPERVISION

Here are some tips for filling in the gaps. During passing period, it's okay if supervisors provide a "visual hand off" rather than escorting a student. As the student leaves classroom A, the teacher for that room stands in the hallway and watches the student walk toward his or her next class. At the corner, teacher B stands outside his classroom and visually signifies to teacher A that he can see the student, and watches as the student enters classroom C where teacher C stands ready to receive.

It is also possible to have the student transition between classes when the hallways are empty, either just before or just after passing period. If a student can't be trusted to comply with either of these scenarios then they may require an escort.

Bathroom breaks can often present a complication to supervision. Generally, there are a few easy solutions here as well. First, a student who cannot use the restroom with peers may benefit from having access to a staff restroom instead. Second, this student should have certain specific times of the day when a restroom break can be accommodated, thereby minimizing the likelihood that her or she will use restroom time as a mechanism for harming others sexually, and helping to establish a routine that your school staff can easily monitor.

Recess can seem like a very difficult environment in which to provide supervision to students. There are countless nooks and crannies on most recess fields, and a number of hiding spots that complicate supervision. Again, these problems can generally be easily overcome by prohibiting play in hard-to-supervise areas, and/or by breaking the recess area up into supervised "zones" and limiting play to those domains that are easiest to supervise. Ultimately though, it may be the case that some kids need to have a closely supervised recess that occurs in a very limited area. Use your best judgment and consult with your multidisciplinary team if you are uncertain how restrictive you need to be.

You can use a similar approach to providing supervision in cafeteria settings as well. Students in need of additional supervision might be better served if they have an assigned seat for lunch at a table near a "knowledgeable adult supervisor." Be mindful that problematic sexual behavior can often occur under the cafeteria table, so encouraging students to keep their hands above the table may assist your supervision.

You can also limit student access to areas of your building. For example, if you have an area that is particularly difficult to supervise, or if you have an unusually vulnerable population in a specific area of your school (think on-campus day care, or SPED room with severely cognitively delayed students), you can bar the student from entering those areas of your school.

ARM'S-REACH SUPERVISION

Having covered most of what you need to know when thinking about "line-of-sight" supervision, let's turn our discussion to "arm's-reach" supervision. "Arm's-reach" supervision is suggested when you believe you need to be able to physically block a student from sexually touching others. In other words, you need to reach out and touch them before they can reach out and touch someone else.

A student may benefit from "arm's-reach" supervision if he is remarkably impulsive or unusually predatory with regard to his sexual behavior. This type of student may require "one-on-one" supervision, reductions in the length of their school day, or more restrictive environments in order to protect staff, community, and peers. Thankfully, these types of students are relatively rare.

KNOWLEDGEABLE ADULT SUPERVISORS

Ok, a bit about knowledgeable adult supervisors. A "knowledgeable adult supervisor" is simply a designated adult who has been informed about the student's need for supervision. This person should NOT be given a detailed history of the student's problematic sexual behavior, but they should know enough about the student and the situation to be able to provide good supervision.

One way to handle this delicate balance is to be thoughtful about the language you use to describe these students and their problems. Use the term "interpersonal boundary issues" to refer to the types of problems that you want your "knowledgeable adult supervisors" to be on the lookout for.

The term *interpersonal boundary issues* could mean that Billy pokes kids in the eye when he gets close to them, or it could mean that Suzy tries to put her hand down her neighbor's pants when she's standing next to them in line. It is a term that is relatively ambiguous but also specific enough to ensure that most "knowledgeable adult supervisors" know what they are supervising for.

You may need to provide your "knowledgeable adult supervisors" additional information as a function of the specifics of the situation. For example, you may have a student who targets younger kids, or one that targets females, or one that targets staff, or one that only engages in problematic sexual behavior while on recess, and so on. The important thing to remember is to include enough information to ensure that the supervisors can do their job without giving them so much information that you have compromised the reputation of your student.

The great thing about having a team of "knowledge adult supervisors" tracking a specific student is not only does it increase safety and help to minimize liability, but it also allows you to gain immediate feedback regarding how well your supervision/intervention plan is working so that you can adjust it accordingly. It also provides you with an ongoing assessment regarding how the student is responding to supervision so that you can determine if the student is actively following the supervision plan or attempting to undermine it.

WATCHING THE WATCHERS

Speaking of students who seek to undermine your supervision plan—it's important to have your "knowledgeable adult supervisors" be on the lookout for students who "watch the watchers." "Watching the watchers," or "opportunistically vigilant" as it is noted on the Level 1 protocol, is a phrase used to describe students who appear to be looking for opportunities to harm others sexually. These students appear to be on the lookout for gaps in supervision and will take advantage of transition times and other more chaotic parts of the day to engage in sexually harmful behavior.

Students who watch the watchers stand out because they seem to be spending as much time supervising you as you are supervising them. Clearly, when you have a student who is engaging in these types of behaviors, it's a sign that you need to have a tight supervision plan that provides him or her little opportunity to harm others.

OTHER SCHOOL-BASED SUPERVISION STRATEGIES

Sometimes students engage in problematic sexual behavior during classroom time. For these students, an assigned seat near supervision and away from potential targets may be very helpful. If you have a student who seems to be targeting females, you can surround his or her desk with a barrier of male students. If you have a student who is touching others during circle time, you can assign a seat near the teacher. Or if you have a student who is sexually targeting a staff member, you can have the student's assigned seat be away from that individual.

Your supervision plan should also include activities that occur on campus after school is in session, like band practice, clubs, sports, and other events like school dances. For some of these events, like sports, accommodations may have to be made regarding where a student changes clothes, or in what kinds of activities they can engage. For example, you probably don't want to encourage someone with problematic sexual behavior to go out for the wrestling team because this is a high-contact sport. Also, you may have to be very thoughtful about swim practice as supervision in a swimming pool can be particularly challenging.

Give thought as well as to who needs to know what about the student in various settings. You'll want to make sure that your band director knows if he has a student in band who has a history of sexually harming female students. If you are allowing a student with problematic sexual behavior to attend a dance, you'll also want to make sure that this does not become a venue in which the student can sexually abuse others. It's not rocket science. Just use common sense and clearly articulate in writing who is responsible for providing supervision in which settings and you can rest assured in your decision-making.

ACADEMIC RESTRICTIONS

Clearly, general education students with problematic sexual behavior do not belong in a classroom with any vulnerable population. These students can't act as student aids in a SPED classroom, they can't work in the school-based day care facility, and they shouldn't be taking classes on childcare. You may also want to limit their involvement in 4H Clubs, or other classes that involve working with animals. Squicky to think about, but you have to consider these things.

Just so you know, evidence suggests that a good chunk of individuals with problematic sexual behavior target animals. Further, you may also want to limit access to technology depending upon their presentation. A student who downloads pornography, or who uses the Internet to groom fellow students should not be allowed computer access.

SPECIAL EDUCATION AND 504 CONSIDERATIONS

It's not unusual to find that a little over half of the students who require supervision plans for problematic sexual behavior come from SPED or have a 504 plan. What this means is that you should always include a SPED or 504 representative (depending upon the student) when establishing a supervision plan. You may need to review the student's IEP or 504 plan before you final-ize your supervision plan. It is important that you follow the law and protect the rights of these students, while also developing a plan that protects your school.

FAMILY ROLE

It is very important that the parents of a student with problematic sexual behavior be made fully aware of the serious liability they need to manage with regard to their child's problematic sexual behavior. They should be made aware that they need to provide for the safety of the other children they have in their home, and they should be referred to a mental health provider in the area who works with kids with problematic sexual behavior.

Most importantly, parents need to understand that once they have the knowledge that their child may be (notice use of the words *may be* . . . you don't need proof, just a reasonable belief) engaging in sexually harmful behavior, they have the legal responsibility to protect others from harm.

Think of it like this. If you had a dog that had a history of biting people, you would need to take special precautions when taking that dog out of the house. Failure to do so is not only immoral and socially irresponsible but also legally liable. If someone were minding his own business, walking down the street and was bitten by this naughty dog, he'd have grounds for a substantial lawsuit against you as legally liable owner. The same is true for the potential victims of child who has been identified as having sexually harmful behavior.

What this means is that parents have the responsibility for informing anyone who supervises their child about this potential liability. Parents should be strongly encouraged to inform the following people and groups about their child's problematic sexual behavior.

- Church officials where their family attends
- Sunday school teacher where their family attends
- Babysitters
- Afterschool programs
- Tutoring programs
- Intramural sports coaches
- Parents who are supervising playdates
- Any adult who provides supervision to their child

Parents are responsible for providing enough information to these individuals to enable them to provide adequate supervision for the purpose of limiting harm to others. Depending upon the situation, it may be prudent to discourage parents from allowing their child to participate in or host sleepovers, and it may be wise to encourage parents to make sure that their child does not share a bedroom with siblings or to set up other safety measures, such as door alarms, hall cameras, and so forth.

The important thing to remember is that the safety plan should *reasonably* address the safety concerns. A child who repeatedly "pees in the barkdust on the playground" should not have the same safety plan as a child who is intentionally targeting disenfranchised peers for sexual victimization.

It is important to document that you have informed the parents of your recommendations and given them a referral to a mental health provider in the area who specializes in working with kids with problematic sexual behavior. Once you have documented this, you have handed off this chunk of liability to the parents. Make sure they understand the potential repercussions for failing to follow through. (Yay! Do your little liability dance. This is one less thing you have to worry about.)

It is now the parents' job to communicate this important information to the community. If the parents fail to follow through with their responsibility, your next step would be to contact Child Protection Services to make them aware of your concerns.

LAW ENFORCEMENT AS INTERVENTION

This is often a hard sell to some educators. Although in recent years educators have become somewhat more comfortable working with law enforcement since the inclusion of school resource officers on school campuses, there persists some hesitancy in many school officials to involve law enforcement with regard to problematic sexual behavior.

It may be that this reluctance stems from the fear that the child will be labeled a sex offender if law enforcement gets involved. This is a realistic fear. If a child has transgressed the law with regard to sexual behavior, he or she may face very real charges, jail time, the possibility of being tried as an adult, and being labeled as a sex offender. It's very serious business, and many administrators think "I don't want to ruin this kid's life over a single incident."

Taking all that into account, here is why you should involve law enforcement, and encourage legal accountability whenever possible. First, involving law enforcement is a mechanism for spreading liability and demonstrating to the community your commitment to safety. When you involve law enforcement, you bring a different skill set to the table, and you start to extend the decision-making and liability outside of your office and into the community. You also send a clear message to your community that you take safety very seriously.

The second reason to involve law enforcement is that they may have access to information you do not. Sure, it seemed like a little innocent sexual touching out on the playground, nothing to report to the police. But would your opinion change if you learned from law enforcement that there had been three previous complaints filed against that student for sexual touching that occurred in the community?

Most individuals with problematic sexual behavior are acting out in a variety of ways in a variety of environments. Generally speaking, the incident that brings their problematic sexual behavior to the attention of others is the tip of the iceberg. By involving law enforcement, there is a good chance you might get a better picture of what lies beneath the surface.

The third, and probably most important reason to involve law enforcement is that, for most individuals with problematic sexual behavior, the only way they will be able to access treatment and assessment is via the legal system. Call up your health-care provider, or query with the state-funded health-care system in your area and ask them how many sessions of sex offender-specific therapy they pay for. The answer is zero. In fact, many states have enacted specific laws to prohibit state funds from being used to treat "behavioral problems" like problematic sexual behavior. It's stupid and fiscally shortsighted, but it's reality.

What this means is that the only way most families can afford to get treatment is via programs that are funded by the legal system. The only way into that system is via adjudication. So, the reality is that law enforcement is your best opportunity to enable a student to get help for serious sexual behavior.

WHEN DOES SUPERVISION DROP?

Unlike supervision plans for students with threatening or potentially concerning violent behavior, which can typically be reduced after the student evidences positive changes with regard to behavior, supervision plans for kids with problematic sexual behavior need to stay in place until there is considerable evidence from multiple sources that a reduction in supervision is recommended.

There are two reasons why it is important to proceed with more caution when reducing supervision for kids with problematic sexual behavior. First, these kids generally don't present with a host of behavioral concerns. They tend to be very careful and cautious about how they act and may even present as particularly well behaved in an attempt to hide their problematic sexual behavior. So, linking a reduction in supervision to behavioral factors is challenging because their baseline behaviors are typically pretty good.

The other reason why it is important to make thoughtful and gradual reductions in supervision is because kids with problematic sexual behavior will often put tremendous effort into managing their persona specifically for the purpose of encouraging a reduction in supervision, so that they can again reengage in harming others sexually.

Here's how it often works. Kevin was exposed to sexual material when he was very young. It created some confusion/anxiety/excitement/curiosity in him that he attempts to relieve by touching others sexually. In a way, it's like an attempt to gain mastery over this troubling thing that he doesn't really understand about himself. It feels bad and good at the same time. Kevin knows this behavior is not okay, and he fears getting caught, so he is especially well behaved in an attempt to distract himself and others from his problematic sexual behavior.

After a while, Kevin gets caught and put on a supervision plan. This makes him very anxious, which makes him want to engage in problematic sexual behavior even more, so that he can relieve tension. He then turns up the notch on his good behavior in the hopes that this might lead to a reduction in supervision, so that he can get back to touching others sexually.

One really easy way to handle reductions in supervision is to move forward with reductions only with the guidance and signed approval of a mental health professional. Relying upon the signed recommendations of a mental health professional to reduce supervision is a good idea because the mental health professional is the only one who has insight into, and the ability to impact, intent.

Relying upon a mental health professional also accomplishes three things. First, it hands the liability off to the therapist, which helps to protect your district. Two, it enables the district to join with the family rather than appear adversarial. It is no longer a district decision when to reduce supervision, but one that lives with the therapist. Three, it encourages families to seek professional help to address problematic sexual behavior in their kids, because the method to reduce supervision is linked directly to treatment.

It is important to note that just because a mental health professional endorses a reduction in supervision does not mean that your district needs to comply. Ultimately, the administrator of every school building is responsible for the safety of the students and staff in that environment, so if the recommendations of the mental health professional seem misguided, don't follow them. One of the ironies here is that any mental health professional who eagerly signs off on a reduction of supervision probably shouldn't be practicing mental health. Clearly, supervision reductions have very serious implications on the health and welfare of the community, so if a therapist doesn't seem to have any sense to the seriousness of these decisions, don't trust him or her.

WHAT IF PARENTS/STUDENTS/STAFF WON'T COMPLY WITH THE SUPERVISION PLAN?

I'm sure in your district parents, students, and staff always comply with your suggestions immediately. I can hear the sound of your eye muscles straining as you fight the urge to roll them. Let's be honest, increased supervision sucks.

Supervision sucks for the kids because it keeps them from engaging in a behavior that they want to engage in. It sucks for the parents because no matter how delicate and deliberate you are in constructing your supervision plan, the parents will see the need for supervision as an endorsement that their child is fundamentally flawed in some way. And it sucks for the school because you now have to implement yet another unfunded plan that involves training staff and juggling your staffing patterns.

Regardless of how much it sucks, however, these plans need to be implemented for community safety, and accountability is the only means of ensuring that these things get followed. So, when resistance occurs, it needs to be addressed immediately and directly. School staff need to understand that failure to follow supervision plans could lead to disciplinary action. Students need to understand that failure to follow the supervision plan could lead to more restrictions and tighter supervision. And families need to know that not following the supervision plan could lead to DHS involvement.

Chapter 7

The Level 2 Team

Sound the trumpets!! It's time to learn about the Level 2 team. Before we get into a detailed discussion, let me give you three bits of information about the Level 2 team. The first important thing to remember about the Level 2 team is that its only job is to act as a consultation team to your school and community.

As a consultation team, this group has no power to enforce or execute. Their sole purpose is to act as a "think tank" that makes thoughtful recommendations to the school and community regarding the supervision of individuals with problematic sexual behavior. For your edification, a visual flowchart of the Level 2 process is included in appendix C.

The second important thing to know is that although the Level 2 team lacks executive power, their recommendations remain incredibly important. Although it is totally within their purview, most administrators and community agencies are reluctant to go against the recommendations of a team of recognized professionals for liability reasons. Consequently, even though there is no executive capacity in the Level 2 team, the recommendations that come out of this process maintain relevance as a result of where and how they originate.

Although this chapter is dedicated to outlining what this team should look like and how it should function, the third important thing to remember is that you can adapt this team to fit your community and your needs. This chapter will provide some ideas about how to do that, and you'll have to pick through those ideas to create a method that works for your system.

TEAM MEMBERS

The Level 2 team should serve the school and community, and it should contain individuals who have expertise in the management of individuals with problematic sexual behavior. Toward that goal, here are some of the recommended players:

- Level 2 facilitator
- Law enforcement/school resource officer
- Juvenile justice staff
- Juvenile parole/probation officers who manage sex offenders
- Community mental health providers
- DHS/Child Protective Services worker
- District attorney's representative
- School counselor/behavioral specialist
- SPED/504 representative
- School psychologist
- School security representative
- Individual/s with expertise in assessment/supervision of individuals with problematic sexual behavior
- Other community liaisons

Please keep in mind that you don't need a separate individual for each role. For example, it may be the case that your school psychologist is the Level 2 facilitator and also your SPED representative. Your school counselor may also act as your 504 representative, and it may be the case that you draw upon multiple sources for expertise with regard to the assessment and supervision of individuals with problematic sexual behavior.

The important thing to keep in mind is that everyone needs to know what their role is in the meeting, what expertise they bring to the table and for whose interests they are advocating. It's also important that everyone understand that the Level 2 team is not solely an arm of the school, but that its mission is to serve the interest of safety across multiple contexts including community and home.

THE LEVEL 2 FACILITATOR

When you think about it, running a successful Level 2 meeting is no easy task. You have a room full of people with differing training and backgrounds. These folks all have different perspectives regarding how best to deal with problematic sexual behavior.

Some people will want to "lock 'em up and throw away the key," while others will demand that "kids get better if you love them enough." Now add to that the fact that as a group you are going to be discussing graphic sexual behavior. It's important that you take a moment to think about this when you are trying to find your facilitator.

Although it's possible to operate a Level 2 team with a revolving chair, given the complexity of the work and its potential impact on community and school safety, the team will function more effectively with a clearly delineated facilitator. It's much easier for everyone involved if there is a single person whose job it is to run the Level 2 meeting and who also acts as a liaison between the Level 1 and Level 2 teams.

In a perfect world, this person would belong to the school district that hosts the Level 2 team. This individual would have a solid understanding of the workings of school districts. He or she would have knowledge of SPED and 504 laws, and would understand what resources school districts have at their disposal. Additionally, this person would also have knowledge about problematic sexual behavior.

Clearly, you can't find all this in one person, so identifying training opportunities and materials will be helpful. A great place to get training with regard to sexually concerning behavior is via the Association for the Treatment of Sexual Behavior (ATSA). ATSA has reading materials to recommend, holds yearly national conferences, publishes their own materials, and most states have ATSA affiliates that offer regular trainings. You can find them online at www.atsa.com. Another great resource is the National Center on the Sexual Behavior of Youth (NCSBY). You can find out more about NCSBY at www .ncsby.org.

In order for the system to work properly, the facilitator will need to understand all the moving parts and how they function. This person needs to understand what a Level 1 and Level 2 meeting should look like. He or she needs to understand how these two teams communicate with each other and he or she needs to understand how schools, communities, law enforcement, and juvenile justice systems interact with one another.

Overseeing and maintaining the system means doing a lot of trainings initially. The facilitator will need to train administrators and school counselors on how to conduct a Level 1 meeting. It will also be important to train Level 1 team members on some basics about how to use the two-level system, problematic sexual behavior, normative sexual behavior in children, school-based supervision strategies, what it means to be a knowledgeable adult supervisor and so forth. Given job turnover and employment changes, these trainings will need to occur on a regular (probably yearly) basis.

At first, the facilitator will probably need to attend a number of Level 1 meetings until team members understand their roles and become more comfortable with how the system functions. You'll also find that you'll want to have the facilitator attend some Level 1 meetings if you anticipate the meeting will be "hot." It's perfectly reasonable to include the facilitator in a meeting where you think the parents may be hostile, or where the sexual behavior is so remarkable or unusual that you feel you need help discussing it. As Level 1 teams become more confident and competent, you can start to phase out facilitator attendance.

The facilitator will also need to craft a mechanism for capturing all the Level 1 and Level 2 data. While it would be impossible for the facilitator to review every Level 1 document, it does make sense that the facilitator (or his or her administrative assistant) review them periodically to ensure fidelity to the model. Also, given the richness of this data, it makes sense to have a way of gathering this information for use by the district. Whether this means creating an online database version of the Level 1 protocol, or getting an interested psychology graduate student to help collect data, it might be wise to, at the very least, make sure you have a central warehouse for all this useful information you will be collecting.

The facilitator will also be responsible for training and maintaining the Level 2 team and helping to encourage community partners to maintain involvement. This will mean hosting some trainings on the Level 2 process and also being willing to go out to the community partners and offer trainings on aspects of the system and on supervising individuals with problematic sexual behavior.

Although the Level 1 protocol does an excellent job of capturing information about a problematic sexual incident, it is not designed to capture all the information you might want about a particular student or case. Consequently, it is recommended that once a referral is made to the Level 2 team, the facilitator gather additional information from the Level 1 team prior to bringing the case to the Level 2 team. There is a form at the back of this book in appendix D that provides an example of the data gathering tool used by Salem-Keizer Public Schools when their facilitator goes data gathering.

The purpose of this data gathering is to answer most of the typical questions about the students that will first be addressed in the Level 2 meeting. Are they in SPED or General Ed? What inhibitors and protective factors exist that might discourage them from engaging in problematic sexual behavior? How are they doing academically? What is their attendance like? Do they like school? Do they have friends? Are those friends a positive or negative influence? How do they deal with stress and upset? What is their general attitude toward authority? Are they on any medications? What is their family system like?

Generally, the data gathering occurs at the school with the school counselor and/or the administrator, just prior to the Level 2 meeting. Sometimes you can choose to skip this step in the event that the Level 1 team decides they are able to attend the Level 2 meeting. But on the whole, it's recommended that the facilitator take some time to gather this information prior to the Level 2 meeting. You will not be able to answer all the questions on the investigation form, but doing your best to complete this form will make your Level 2 meeting run more efficiently because it provides the Level 2 team a much deeper understanding of the individual and how best to intervene.

Finally, the facilitator will be responsible for reporting Level 2 recommendations back to the Level 1 team. There is a form in appendix D designed to be used in this capacity as well as a letter that can accompany the Inquiry Summary when sending the Level 2 recommendations on to the Level 1 team.

FACILITATION OF THE LEVEL 2 TEAM

The primary job of the facilitator is to inspire and help steer conversation during the Level 2 meeting. Although a detailed description of how the Level 2 meeting works follows in the next chapter, it's worth taking a few moments to address facilitation generally here.

During the Level 2 meeting, the facilitator is somewhat akin to an orchestra conductor. While the goal of a music conductor is to pull an inspiring and organized performance out of musicians, the goal of the Level 2 facilitator is to pull inspired supervision planning and interventions out of a multidisciplinary team of professionals. Like the orchestra conductor, the Level 2 facilitator must work to eliminate noise (cacophony) and work to bring balance to the piece (harmony).

PEOPLE YOU NEED TO THINK CAREFULLY
ABOUT BEFORE INCLUDING

While there may be some value to having a local sex offender treatment provider sitting on your team, this may create a significant conflict of interest because it complicates the referral process. You can't ethically send all your Level 2 kids to your own team member for treatment or further assessment, so if you do decide to include a treatment provider (or if you have to have a treatment provider on your team because there are so few individuals with expertise in your region), please be very explicit regarding how referrals will be handled so as not create a conflict of interest.

As a rule, parents should not be allowed to participate in the Level 2 meeting. Again, the purpose of the Level 2 is so the community and school can access expertise on safety planning and evenly distribute liability. The Level 2 meeting is a domain in which professionals need to be able to have very candid discussions for the purpose of protecting the community at large.

Including a parent in the Level 2 discussion will limit the candor with which these issues can be addressed. Further, there really is no reason why a parent should ever have any need to attend. They can provide input into the process via the Level 1 team should they chose to do so.

While representatives from the DA's office should be encouraged to attend Level 2 meetings if possible, there really is no reason to have additional legal representation from other agencies at the table. If one agency brings a lawyer, then all agencies will want to have one there as well, which will make the cost of running such an endeavor prohibitive.

TO WHOM DOES THE LEVEL 2 TEAM BELONG?

Ideally, the Level 2 team should belong to a school district or educational service district. More than any organization, the school district directly benefits from the consultation provided by the Level 2 team, so it makes sense to house it under their roof. Kids spend more time at school than in any other domain, and more and more (much to the chagrin of our embarrassingly underfunded schools) schools function as the center point for connecting families to community resources. As such, schools are perfectly positioned to serve as the host of the Level 2 team. As such, schools are perfectly positioned to serve as the host of the Level 2 team.

The aforementioned having been considered, however, there is no reason why the Level 2 team couldn't be hosted by the Department of Juvenile Justice (DA's office or Parole and Probation), law enforcement, the DHS (Child Protective Services), or an independent community-based group concerned with public safety. All these other agencies have a significant stake in the supervision of kids with problematic sexual behavior, so these other agencies can easily serve as host as well.

HOW DO YOU GET ALL THESE PEOPLE TOGETHER?

A good Level 2 team can only be developed by partnering with community stakeholders. In some environments where there have been solid long-standing relationships between agencies, this can be as simple as calling a meeting of all the interested parties and ironing out the logistics. In communities where the relationships are unestablished or unhealthy, creating a Level 2 may take more work.

If you are working in a community where there are systemic issues, you may want to begin by enlisting the help of a neutral third party. For example, let's say that there is poor communication between law enforcement and the school district, but that both parties have a good relationship with juvenile justice. It may be that juvenile justice can act as a sort of Switzerland in this situation by helping other agencies reach a common ground. It can also be very helpful to have a Level 2 facilitator who is adept at connecting with people; someone who enjoys being at the center of things; a social butterfly of sorts.

Clearly, this team cannot be constructed without considerable effort. But just like every long journey begins with a single step, so does every success- ful Level 2 team start with a single meeting. Start with agencies with whom you partner well, get them on board, then use those connections to help you build relationships with the agencies you don't know as well or have had trouble with in the past.

HIPAA/FERPA, MEMORANDUMS OF UNDERSTANDING, AND CONFIDENTIALITY

Many people wonder, if they are even allowed to discuss specific information about students given the limits of HIPAA and FERPA? You'll be happy to learn that HIPAA (Health Insurance Portability and Accountability Act) and FERPA both have clauses in them that allow for interagency communication without prior consent when matters of public safety are at hand.

Now, speak to a few lawyers about this, and you'll find their take is that "public safety" is a very fuzzy line with regard to problematic sexual behavior. While it's very easy to justify that agencies be allowed free com- munication without prior consent when there is a potential school shooter on the prowl, it's another thing entirely to attempt to use this clause as a justification for sharing information when the discussion is about problem- atic sexual behavior. The threat of harm is generally not as imminent, the target not as clearly articulated, and the scope of the threat is typically not as significant.

All that being said, many lawyers take the position that they would much rather be in court defending an agency from allegations of unauthorized infor- mation sharing that was intended to protect the safety of the community, than they would trying to defend that same agency from allegations that they could have done more to warn potential targets of an impending sexual threat that resulted in real victimization. Ultimately, you'll want to talk to your school district lawyers to determine where they are most comfortable in regard to the issue of information sharing.

Keeping all that in mind, there are some things that you can do in order to better enable interagency communication without violating HIPAA/FERPA. One thing you can do is acquire a release of information (ROI) from the parents of every individual that is captured by your Level 1 process before taking anything to a Level 2. When a parent comes in for the Level 1, you collect the needed signatures during that meeting that allows information sharing between the various agencies.

Be warned, this may slow down your process and create other sorts of problems. What happens if the parent refuses to sign the release? Do you make signing the release contingent before the student can return to school? How will you acquire the release (and how long will it take) if the parent doesn't show up for the Level 1? You will want to have answers for these questions before you decide to go this route, and you'll probably want to look at your district's policies and procedures, and consult with legal counsel so that you know how firm a stance you can take with this approach.

Using memorandums of understanding (MOU) is another tack you can take to help solve this problem. MOU's (sometimes called memorandums of agreement) are contracts that exist between agencies that enable them to have free and open discussions regarding individuals, provided that the information remains confidential and is not shared outside of that meeting.

There is an example of the MOU used by Salem-Keizer Public Schools at the back of this book in appendix F. If you plan to go this route (which is recommended), you'll want to run this document by your legal counsel, as will all the other agencies signing it. This will likely take some time, and you do not want to sign off on the MOU until all agencies have agreed to the wording in the document.

Be warned, the complicating factor in using MOUs is that it's very hard to add new members to your group once everyone has signed their MOUs because every time you do, every agency needs to sign another MOU that includes that newest agency. Arggh!

To be on the safe side, it's also important to have anyone attending the Level 2 meeting sign a confidentiality agreement before being allowed to attend. That means that you will have all your regular members sign a confidentiality agreement when they first join the group and then you will need to make sure that any visitors to your meeting or new individuals sign a confidentiality agreement before any discussion occurs. You'll find an example of the one used by Salem-Keizer at the back of this book in appendix F.

WHAT HAPPENS AT A LEVEL 2 MEETING?

For the first few months, the facilitator will want to begin every meeting with introductions. It never ceases to amaze me how frequently people fail to follow this simple social convention. But given the importance of establishing trust and good working relationship between your partners, it is vital that everyone at the table know who is at the table and from which agencies they hail. Once members have gotten to know each other, it will only be important to remember to do introductions when new members or guests show up.

After introductions, the facilitator will want to make sure that any new members or guests have filled out the confidentiality agreement before beginning the discussion. Once this is taken care of, you can move to a discussion of any important business before addressing cases.

When discussing business, Level 2 members can bring in topics that have bearing on the functioning of the Level 2 team or that might be of interest to the group. This should include any changes in scheduling, meeting locations, and things of that sort. Also, a good facilitator will use this time to bring up important information relevant to the understanding of problematic sexual behavior. For example, this could include informing the team about important trainings or conferences about problematic sexual behavior, or keeping the team abreast of the latest research or publications in the area.

After discussing business, the facilitator presents the cases one by one and leads the team in a case-by-case discussion aimed at addressing the supervision and safety needs of the various Level 1 referrals. Ideally, it is advantageous to have members from the referring Level 1 team present at the Level 2 case presentation and discussion. If this is not possible, then the facilitator takes responsibility for case presentation.

During the case presentation, Level 2 team members should be encouraged to ask questions and provide their thoughts about the situation, and the facilitator should bring to light any specific concerns that encouraged the Level 1 team to bring the case to the Level 2 team. From there, the facilitator leads the Level 2 team in a discussion toward the goal of developing specific recommendations designed to increase safety and intervene in the problematic sexual behavior. After the team develops their recommendations, the team sets a date to further review the case for the purpose of assessing progress (there's your ongoing assessment piece, pretty cool, huh?).

Either the facilitator or an appointed secretary takes notes regarding the details of the discussion and the recommended disposition for each case, including any assigned duties as a result of the discussion. This note taker will then e-mail a list of duties out to the Level 2 team members so that all members are aware of who is responsible for taking specific actions. These actions will be followed up on during the next discussion of the case.

After all the cases have been discussed, the facilitator closes the meeting and makes contact with all the referring Level 1 teams to provide them an immediate synopsis of the case recommendations. The facilitator then generates a report for each Level 2 referral that was discussed and sends those reports to the Level 1 teams shortly after the meeting (ideally no longer than a week). You'll find an example of a Level 2 report at the end of the book.

EXAMPLE

Just for fun, let's look at a brief example of how a Level 2 meeting might function if Amanda from the previous chapter was referred for a Level 2.

After going over introductions and addressing business concerns, the facilitator begins with a presentation of Amanda's case. The facilitator, we'll call her Tracey, is aided in the presentation by Amanda's school counselor (Kevin) and administrator (Jason), both of whom are deeply concerned about Amanda's sexual behavior:

Tracey (facilitator): "The basics of the case are as follows. Amanda is a third grader at Van Dreal Elementary School. She's been on the radar for some time due to poor boundaries around adult men and problems with sexual talk and touching her peers. Recently, however, things have gotten more serious. I'll let Kevin explain."

Kevin (school counselor): "Last week our first grade teacher Ms. Goss became concerned when one of the students she sent to the restroom had not returned. When Ms. Goss went to check on her student, she discovered Amanda and her student with their pants down around their ankles. Amanda was on her knees and had inserted her finger into the other girl's vagina. Ms. Goss was shocked, to say the least, and told the girls to get dressed. She then brought them to me and Jason."

Jason (administrator): "The first grader, Kim, was immediately forthcoming and described that Amanda had told her during recess to ask to go to the bathroom when she got back to class from recess. Kim said that Amanda told her to pull her pants down and also not to tell or she would get into trouble. Kim seemed more confused than upset."

Kevin: "Amanda was another story altogether. She denied the entire incident ever happened and was steadfast in her resolve. It didn't matter how many different ways I tried to get at what happened. Nice guy, tough guy, she didn't crack."

Tracey: "Okay. What questions does the group have?"

Becky (school resource officer): "Do we have any history on Amanda or her family?"

Kevin: "The family lives in an apartment complex about half a mile from the school. It's not the nicest place, but certainly not the worst either. We don't see the mom a whole lot, but the dad comes in almost every week. I wouldn't describe him as involved; he doesn't do much to help out, never volunteers in the classrooms, but he does check in pretty regularly to see how Amanda is doing."

Becky: "Do we have a name and DOB [date of birth] on the dad?"

Jason: "His name is Jim Martini. I don't have a DOB but I'd say he's in his late twenties."

Becky: "I'll see what I can find" (Becky leaves the room briefly to look up information on Jim Martini).

Andrea (SPED consultant): "What can you tell us about Amanda generally, academics, socialization, etc. Is she a SPED kid?"

Kevin: "Not SPED yet, but Amanda doesn't have many friends her age. Most of her classmates steer clear of her. At recess she mostly plays with younger kids. She's pretty immature on some levels, but in other ways very precocious. I make it a point to always leave my door open or have another adult with me when I meet with her because she has very poor boundaries. I know this sounds weird, but sometimes she almost seems flirtatious. First time I met her, she tried to get up in my lap. Academically, she's an average student. She comes across as pretty distracted in class, but seems to be holding her own academically. Most of the difficulty she has is interpersonal. She lies a great deal and often gets upset because she can't get her peers to interact with her."

Becky: "Hey just got a hit on the name Jim Martini. Thirty-one-year-old male, looks like he grew up in California. He's got a sexual misconduct charge there that happened when he was eighteen. I don't have the details of it, but will put a call in to the department later today to request the arrest report. Looks like he's not on the sex offender registry, but sometimes these things get dropped when people leave the state. I'll do a little more poking around and let you know what I come up with as things develop."

Alan (county mental health): "Mom wouldn't happen to be Alice Martini would it?"

Jason: "Yes. That's her mom."

Alan: "I can't provide any information about the mom, but I can tell you that Alice has brought another girl, Debbie I think, into see us on three occasions. Does Amanda have a sister?"

Jason: "No."

Alan: "Hmmm. What does Amanda look like?"

Jason: "Let me pull up a photo of her."

Alan: "Yeah. That's her. I met with her twice. When I saw her she appeared pretty distressed and anxious. A little shell-shocked. She wouldn't reveal anything... wouldn't talk to me much at all. Left me with a very unsettled feeling, but I didn't have anything tangible to file a report with DHS. Alice told me the girl's name was Debbie. Looks like things are starting to get a bit more complicated."

Tracey: "Agreed. I think we may have some ideas about where this could be headed. But let's not jump to conclusions yet. When you hear a stampede it's probably horses... but sometimes it's zebras. Let's see what other data we have. Also, I'd like to hear about the school's supervision needs."

Jason: "We've got her on a pretty tight watch. We don't have the resources to give her a one-on-one and one of the things we were hoping to get the Team's input on is whether or not you think we need one. You can see what we've done in the *supervision plan: changed her classroom seating assignment; she's escorted to the bathroom; the teacher is very careful about transitions now; no more lining up in a free for all; always makes sure to put Amanda near supervision. We've limited her freedom on the playground, and she's using the staff bathroom now, no more regular bathroom for her."*

Tracey: "That all sounds really good. Is she the sort of kid who watches the watchers?"

Kevin: "Oh yeah. She's always got an eye to dips in supervision."

Tracey: "Given that, it will be important to rotate your knowledgeable adult supervisors on a regular basis to prevent fatigue. Also, you'll want to encourage supervisors to be keyed into what she says as well as what she does. They'll need to stay in earshot. This latest situation suggests that Amanda has the sophistication to identify vulnerable kids and the charisma to get them to do what she wants."

Kevin: "She sounds predatory."

Tracey: "I hate to use that terminology, especially on a kid so young. We don't know what we don't know about this case yet. What I would say is that she certainly is determined and clever. We're going to need a particularly tight supervision plan for her. What about community issues? And do the parents seem interested in treatment or getting help for her?"

Jason: "Really hard to say about the parents. The dad came in for the Level 1. Seemed very nervous and was pretty quiet. The only thing he mentioned was that maybe it would be a better idea to take her out of school and homeschool her. We discussed the importance of getting her some support, gave the parents the list of providers, and let them know that we'd continue with the same level of supervision until we had solid evidence from a mental health provider that Amanda could handle less supervision. I'm not holding my breath."

Kevin: "I've heard dad talk about church involvement. I'm not sure if Amanda is plugged into other community supports."

Alan: "Did you make it clear to the parents that they needed to inform the church and other care providers about Amanda's behavior?"

Jason: "Oh yeah. We made it clear and documented it."

Tracey: "Okay. Let's summarize where we are and see what else we need to cover. Becky is looking into the dad. Might be wise to have her look at mom as well, see if there is any history of domestic stuff around the house. Too bad DHS isn't here today. It would have been helpful to get their two cents. I'll call them this afternoon and see what they have to say about this. See if there is an open file, if not, see if they want to open one. As for the school, sounds like you'll make sure our supervisors know to stay within earshot. Other ideas?"

Hopefully, you can see where this meeting is headed as well as how these different players are meant to interact. The goal of the meeting is to gather information from all sources for the purpose of developing a comprehensive plan of action.

As the picture starts to develop, the team will be more certain about how best to respond. But a great deal of the success hangs on the facilitation. The discussion must be focused and direct, and everyone should leave the meeting with a clear understanding of what they need to do.

It's not important that absolutely everything get solved in one meeting. In fact, you will probably need to meet several times over the course of weeks to discuss a case before retiring it. The important thing is that until resolution occurs, your team continues to collect data, and continues to shape the intervention as a function of what they learn. It's a basic empirical process: observe, collect data, develop hypotheses, test hypotheses, observe, collect data, develop new hypotheses, and so on.

Chapter 8

Case Example

Sometimes it can be challenging to understand how all the puzzle pieces fit together, so this chapter is dedicated to following a single case from start to finish, with completed forms and paperwork included at the back of the chapter. Let's get started.

Jennifer is a nine-year-old in the third grade. As a result of some lagging language deficits, she was placed in SPED under speech and language. Although her behavior is good, her academic performance is generally low and there has been some speculation that additional testing might be warranted. Jennifer frequently comes to school looking disheveled, and little is known about her family as she is new to the district. This morning she was discovered in the girl's restroom attempting to digitally penetrate the vagina of Cindy, a girl in her class.

Upon learning of this, the school administrator, Clinton, makes the decision to send Jennifer home and consults with his school counselor, Miguel, to decide what to do. Together they examine page two of the Level 1 protocol (appendix A) to determine if they should conduct a Level 1 meeting.

After reading the criteria, they decide to hold a Level 1 meeting before allowing Jennifer to return to school, and they make the decision to report the incident to law enforcement. Miguel contacts the school resource officer (SRO), Becky, to report the incident and then contacts Jennifer's parents. The Level 1 is set for following morning. Due to the seriousness of the concern, the SRO decides to attend the meeting, as does Angela, Jennifer's SPED case manager.

LEVEL 1

The next morning Jennifer's father, Rick, shows up for the Level 1 meeting. He has Jennifer and her younger sister in tow. The children appear dirty and are very clingy to their father. Miguel finds a task for the children to do, and asks the front desk staff to keep an eye on the girls, while the Level 1 meeting takes place in a separate room.

Clinton (administrator): "Thanks for coming on such short notice."

Rick (father): "Yeah. What's all this about?"

Clinton: "I'll be happy to explain the purpose of this meeting, but before I do, I wanted to make sure that introductions have occurred. Rick, this is Miguel, our school counselor; Becky, our school resource officer; and Angela, Jennifer's special education case manager."

"Yesterday, Jennifer was involved in some behavior at school that we are struggling to understand, and so this morning we are going to go over a protocol that the district uses to help us understand what happened and plan how best to address it. I really appreciate your being here because it makes this process work much better for Jennifer. If no one has any questions, let's get started." (Clinton turns to page three of the Level 1 protocol and reads the information at the top of that page. He then starts the screening portion of the Level 1.)

Let's pick up the discussion on page four when the team begins to examine the incident itself.

Clinton: "Okay. We've got the demographics taken care of. The SRO was notified. Check. Was this determined to be illegal? Becky?"

Becky (SRO): "Well, technically it's a contact offense, so, yes, it's illegal. However, Jennifer is very young, and so, honestly, I'd be very surprised if the DA pursued it. All that being said, I filed a police report that will come to the attention of the DA. So it's in their hands now."

Clinton: "Okay. Rick, what do you know about what happened yesterday?"

Rick: "All I know is what I heard from your counselor. Sounds like she was in the girls' room playing doctor with another girl. I'm not sure why you guys are making such a big deal out of it."

Clinton: "I hear your concern, Rick. In truth, part of the reason we do the Level 1 is to make sure that we don't make too big of a deal out of it. Becky, what information do you have?"

Becky: "It appears that at around 9:30 yesterday morning, Ms. Takahashi discovered Jennifer and a girl from her class in a stall together in the girls' bathroom. Initially, she noticed two sets of legs in the stall and so she approached the stall and opened it, as it was unlocked. She discovered Jennifer on her knees in front of another female student who was sitting on the toilet with her pants down. It appeared to Ms. Takahashi that Jennifer was digitally penetrating the other girl. Ms. Takahashi made sure the girls were dressed and immediately brought them out of the bathroom. She took Jennifer directly to the main office to meet with you, Clinton. The other girl was taken to Miguel's office."

Clinton: "Right. I then asked Jennifer what happened. She reported that the other girl's pants accidentally fell down and that she was helping her to pull them up. She denied touching her genital area. That's when I contacted you, Becky. Miguel?"

Miguel (school counselor): "I spent a little time talking with the other girl. She indicated that she was using the toilet when Jennifer opened the door to her stall and came in. According to her, Jennifer came up to her and said she needed to 'check her pootie,' at which point Jennifer began trying to digitally penetrate her. The little girl I spoke to seemed pretty confused by the whole thing. A little upset. A little grossed out. She kept asking why Jennifer would want to touch where her pee comes out. Mostly she just seemed confused."

Becky: "That's all consistent with my report."

Clinton: "Okay. Thanks. I got all that written down. Let's look at question 1" (reads question 1 aloud)

.Angela (SPED case manager): "Well, they are the same age, but I know that the other girl has some cognitive deficits. We've had some questions in the past about where Jennifer is cognitively, so it's difficult to tell how different they are developmentally. My sense is that the other girl is probably a bit cognitively lower than Jennifer."

Clinton: "Okay. I'm going to mark yes, but I'll include the additional information you shared" (Clinton reads question 2).

Miguel: "I don't have anything in her file, but we're still waiting to receive some information from her last school district. Rick, do you know of anything?"

Rick: "Um. No."

Clinton: "Has she ever engaged in this type of behavior at home? With her siblings? Friends at a sleepover?"

Rick: "No."

Clinton: "Okay. So I guess the answer to number 3 is also no. Let's look at number 4 (reads number 4). Rick, do you know if Jennifer has been exposed to any inappropriate sexual content? Pornography? Maybe an older sibling who talks about sex a lot? Anything?"

Rick: "What are you implying?"

Clinton: "I'm not implying anything. It's just that this is pretty unusual behavior for a child her age and sometimes these things can be the result of a child seeing something that confuses them."

Rick: "We run a good Christian family. None of that stuff goes on in our home."

Clinton: "Do you have any idea where she might have learned this behavior?"

Rick: "No."

Clinton: "Okay. Let's look at question 5. I think we can agree the answer to that is no."

Rick: "Are you saying Jennifer lied? 'Cause I can tell you she isn't a liar. Wasn't raised that way."

Clinton: "Rick. We're not saying that. We're just noting that the stories are different. We don't know what happened. Probably never really will, but we're just trying to do our best to make sense of what happened to make sure it doesn't happen again."

Rick: "Hmm."

Clinton: (Reads question 6) "I don't think we know the answer to that one. Becky?"

Rick: "What's coercion mean?"

Clinton: "Coercion means, did Jennifer try to pressure the other girl in any way?"

Becky: "It's not clear to me that coercion occurred. So I'd mark no."

Clinton: (Reads question 7) "I know from our training that it's pretty unusual for a prepubescent child to engage in sexually penetrative behavior. You wouldn't expect her to have much knowledge about that kind of touching, and it's pretty unusual for a kid her age to have an interest in touching others sexually unless she was exposed to it in some fashion."

Rick: "Are you saying she was molested? 'Cause I can promise you that never happened. I watch her and her sister like a hawk. The only time Jennifer is out of my sight is when she's at school or church."

Clinton: "No, Rick. I'm not implying that. I'm just saying that this behavior is not developmentally normative. Most girls her age don't engage in this type of behavior. If Jennifer is displaying this behavior, it might indicate that she is struggling with something and we'd like to get her help if that is the case."

Rick: "What does that mean? You gonna try to take her away from me? Is that what you mean by help?"

Becky: "Rick. No one is talking about taking Jennifer away from you. We're here to try to find out what this behavior is about so we, all of us Rick, including you and her mom, know best how to help her."

Clinton: "Let's look at number 8. (Reads question 8) I know Jennifer didn't seem particularly upset about it. She seemed more interested in denying it than anything. Miguel, what was your impression of the other girl?"

Miguel: "I don't think she evidenced physical or emotional pain, but she certainly was confused."

Clinton: "Okay. (Reads question 9) I can say that Jennifer didn't have much of an explanation for it. Mostly denied it. Rick, what did Jennifer say when you asked her about it?"

Rick: "I didn't ask her about it. I told her not to talk about it. We have a Christian household. We don't talk about that kinda stuff. It's not right. I told her I didn't want to have that kind of talk in our house."

Miguel: "Rick, I can certainly understand your not wanting to talk about it. These are difficult topics to discuss, especially with kids. But it might really help Jennifer, and it might help all of us if you had a discussion with her about it. It might help all of us adults figure out if Jennifer is in need of help."

Rick: "Look. Those are my kids. I'm not gonna have you telling me about how to raise them. We don't discuss that stuff in our house and that's not about to change. I'm done here. You people can't tell me what to do. Where are my girls?"

Clinton: "Rick, we really need you to stay. You have so much useful information about Jennifer that might really help her. The decisions we make today are important ones and we really want you to be a part of that decision-making process."

Rick: "You're going to make up your own damn decisions to do whatever the hell you want. I'm taking my girls home." (Rick leaves the meeting, grabs his daughters, and leaves the building.)

Angela: "Wow. That went really poorly. I know this is a new family, but does anyone have insight into what's going on there?"

Miguel: "Yeah . . . I know a little something."

Clinton: "I think we get to that in a minute on this protocol. Let's keep working through it. So for number 9 it looks like we don't have much insight into why it happened because Jennifer is largely denying it (reads number 10). Any noticeable difference in physical size or socioeconomic status between these two girls?"

Miguel: "No. They are pretty similar with regard to both. If anything, the other girl comes from a less impoverished home."

Clinton: "Okay. (Reads number 11) I think that is a definite no. What about number 12, grooming? Has Jennifer been paying a lot of undue attention to this other girl?"

Angela: "No. They don't play together. I don't think Jennifer even knows the other girl's name. Jennifer keeps to herself pretty much."

Clinton: "Okay. And the last question. (Reads question 13) Yeah, especially with how the father handled it. I think I'm definitely having a 'strong visceral response.'"

Miguel: "Me too."

Becky: "Yeah."

Clinton: "Okay. Other concerns. We probably won't be able to address many of these. Let's see, would you describe her as planful?"

Miguel: "I really can't say."

Angela: "I'm not sure either."

Clinton: "Impulsive?"

Miguel: "Again. Not sure."

Clinton: "Opportunistically vigilant?"

Miguel: "Remind me what that means again."

Clinton: "Does she watch the watchers?"

Angela: "Yes. I'd say that captures her very well. She does seem to always be keeping an eye on whoever is supervising her."

Clinton: "I don't think we have any evidence of intent to harm self or others or fire set. Miguel, you said you knew a few things about the family. Now would be a great time to share that information."

Miguel: "Like I said, I don't know a whole lot. Dad doesn't work. I think he receives support from Developmental Disabilities. My impression is, he stays home with the kids. Wife works outside the home at a factory job. I think she kinda holds things together. I've never seen the wife before or even spoken to her. It's always the dad. Jennifer doesn't appear to be all that well cared for; sometimes she's a little dirty, but she's certainly not on our radar. We've got other kids who present with much more serious needs. I think the family moved in from Idaho about three or four months ago. We're still waiting to receive a lot of the academic records."

Clinton: "Okay. See if you can contact the counselor at her old school and get more information. See if she's ever done this sort of thing before. See if they know anything about interacting with the family. Do we know if there's been any DHS involvement?"

Becky: "Not since they've been here. I checked before the meeting, but they haven't been here long. I'm going to get on the horn and see if there is anything of interest in Idaho."

Clinton: "That would be great. Okay. Let's finish the protocol and then we can move onto case disposition. The Sexual Behavior Continuum considers this behavior to be of higher concern. I think we're all in agreement (Clinton reads the Level 2 considerations to the team). What do you think? Level 2?"

Miguel: "Definitely."

(Clinton fills out the Level 1 Outcome, transfers the disposition results to page one of the protocol and passes the document around for signatures.)

Clinton: "Okay. Let's get to supervision planning. Intent. We don't know much about this so I'm marking 'engage in problematic sexual behavior.' Target. Looks like female peers. Opportunities . . ." (continues filling out the document).

Clinton: "Who can give me a rundown of Jennifer's day?"

Angela: "I've got that. Her dad drops her off every morning and from there . . ." (Team continues working to develop a supervision plan for Jennifer. You can see the plan they developed at the end of this chapter. After completing the Level 1, Miguel sends the document to the Level 2 facilitator and makes phone contact to schedule the Level 2 inquiry.)

LEVEL 2 INQUIRY

(At the Level 2 inquiry with Miguel and Clinton)

Henry (Level 2 facilitator): "All right, let's get down to it. I recorded the basics from the Level 1. Sounds like you've got a third grade female who digitally penetrated a female peer in the bathroom. Is that correct?"

Clinton: "Yes."

Henry: "Okay. No other students involved but Jennifer and the other girl, motive unclear. How are you guys understanding what happened? What are the circumstances under which this occurred?"

Miguel: "Well, we don't have much information. Jennifer's father walked out of the Level 1 and Jennifer was pretty deceptive regarding her role in what occurred. My sense is there is more to that story."

Henry: "I've got some questions for you about her family. We'll get there in a minute. What about inhibitors?"

Clinton: "Again, we're lacking a lot of information here, but from what I can tell we don't have any evidence that there are any significant inhibitors. Jennifer is pretty much denying anything happened and I'd say her family situation is hardly supportive."

Henry: "How about school? How's Jennifer doing academically?"

Miguel: "From what we can tell, she needs some help. She receives services for speech and there is some speculation that additional testing might be in order. Generally, I'd say she is performing below average in reading and math."

Henry: "How's her attendance?"

Miguel: "Attendance is okay. She was out a few weeks ago for illness. Gone about three days altogether. Not sure what for. Other than that she is generally here."

Henry: "Does she like school?"

Miguel: "Honestly, she seems kind of disorganized. I'm not so sure she really gets that she's at school or not at school. She's not a problem behaviorally, but she doesn't seem really connected either."

Henry: "Any discipline issues?"

Clinton: "No. Other than this incident, not much."

Henry: "Relationship with peers, adults?"

Miguel: "She's pretty new, but like I said, not really connected."

Henry: "Do the other kids avoid her?"

Miguel: "No. She's kind of a new commodity, so to speak. So I don't think the other kids have figured out where she fits."

Henry: "Given that you don't know her very well and her parents aren't participating, we'll skip the section on Personal Factors. What can you tell me about the family?"

Miguel: "Pretty limited. She lives with her parents and her younger sister. Her mom works at a factory job and her dad stays at home with her and her little sister. I can tell you that her father was very resistant to the Level 1, ended up walking out. He appeared less concerned about Jennifer and more concerned that we might be implying he had something to do with it. Very odd. Becky (SRO) is running a background check on him and contacting DHS to see if they have had any concerns at the residence. The dad also seems a little slow, as if he might have some cognitive deficits. Either way, it sounds as if the family is not necessarily going to be on board. Of course, that could look differently if we spoke to Jennifer's mother. Also, sounds as if the family attends church. I'm not sure which one, but that's a potential domain of support."

Henry: "That's also a domain of concern. It's another area in which Jennifer could potentially harm others if she isn't adequately supervised. Hopefully Becky's background check can help us fill in the details. I've got just a few more questions . . . medications, that sort of stuff."

After Henry finishes the Level 2 inquiry, he goes over the preliminary supervision plan developed by the Level 1 team to see if he can make any immediate recommendations. He then examines Jennifer's student records, including her disciplinary information, academic records, and SPED testing so that he can include the relevant information in the inquiry. Unfortunately, with Jennifer being new, and not having her old records on file, his examination of her records turns up very little. On his way out of the school, Henry stops by Becky's (SRO) office to invite her to the Level 2 meeting.

LEVEL 2 MEETING

Two days after the Level 2 inquiry, the Level 2 team meets in a large conference room in the school district main office. In attendance are Henry (Level 2 facilitator), Dustin (deputy from the sheriff's office), Marnie (county mental health specialist), Becky (SRO), Allison (school counselor liaison from school district), Reba (DHS case worker), Seth (head of security from school district), Serena (police officer liaison), Rich (Juvenile Justice probation officer), Michelle (parole officer from Youth Authority), Kathy (school social worker), Steven (liaison from the district attorney's office), Kurt (liaison from Child Sexual Abuse Assessment Unit), and Miguel (school counselor from the referring school).

As Miguel is the only new member to the Level 2 team, Henry has him sign a confidentiality waiver as people are filing in. Henry hands out meeting agendas (that contain a list of all the cases to be discussed and any business that relates to the Level 2 team), leads introductions, takes care of any announcements or business, and then introduces the first case as he passes around the sign-in sheet."

Henry: "Looks like kind of a slow week. We've only got one new case. Jennifer is a nine-year-old third grader at Random Elementary. Earlier this week she was discovered in the girls' bathroom digitally penetrating a female peer. Jennifer is largely in denial about the details of the situation and claims she was trying to help the girl get her pants back up. The other girl appeared very forthcoming about what occurred and said that Jennifer told her she needed to 'examine her pootie.' Miguel, what can you tell us about Jennifer?"

Miguel: "Well, Jennifer is new to the district. We don't have very much on file with regard to her history so I called the school counselor at her last school. The guy wasn't all that helpful, but did indicate that Jennifer had had some issues in kindergarten. Apparently she kept rubbing her groin against her desk at school.

They talked to the parents about it and found out she had a UTI. Apparently, this was an ongoing issue for her at school. Other than that, I didn't get much from him. I can tell you she's in special education for speech and language" (Miguel continues to fill in the Level 2 team with regard to his knowledge of the student).

Henry: "Miguel, could you say a bit about Jennifer's father's presentation during the Level 1."

Miguel: "Yeah, very odd. Obviously, parents are not always happy about having to do a Level 1, but Rick's behavior was very unusual. He was very hostile toward the process and seemed to think we were implying that he had something to do with it. He ended up leaving before the end of the meeting, and he's kept Jennifer out of school since our meeting. He called yesterday to ask what he needed to do in order to homeschool Jennifer."

Becky: "I may be able to shed some light on Rick's behavior. I ran a background check on him. He's got nothing in this state, but he was convicted of a sexual offense in Nevada back in 1992, and served six years in prison for two counts of sodomy. I've requested the records to get more information but from what I can tell it looks like the victim was his six-year-old niece. Upon completing prison, he was remanded to treatment, which it appears he completed along with his parole conditions, and then he was put on the sex offender registry. Now, back in the early 1990s folks were still trying to figure out the sex offender registry in some states, so it's not clear to me if he is still required to be on the sex offender registry in our state. If he is, then we've got a reason to collar him based on that alone. I should have the answer to that by the end of today and I can update the team next week."

Henry: "That's a lot of very helpful information, Becky. Thank you. Okay. This doesn't mean that Rick has done anything to his girls. But it certainly explains some of his cagey behavior. Do we have any reports from DHS?"

Reba (DHS liaison): "In fact we do. About three weeks ago we got an anonymous call indicating that Jennifer was exhibiting some strange behavior at church. According to the caller, Jennifer was found in the church nursery taking off the diaper of a female toddler. When asked what she was doing, Jennifer claimed the toddler told her that her 'pootie hurt' and so she was checking it. The caller remarked that the toddler was not yet verbal. We've sent a worker by the house twice and we've made several calls to the house, but have been unable to reach the parents. The worker we sent said he was pretty sure someone was home when he went by the house but no one answered the door. Our plan was to have law enforcement accompany us on our next visit."

Becky: "I'm getting a bad feeling about this. I'm going to call to see if they can send an officer over to the house right now to do a wellness check. I'll be right back."

Henry: "Thanks, Becky. Okay. Let me give you the remaining rundown on Jennifer from the Level 2 Inquiry and then we can discuss the case (Henry presents the remaining information). Thoughts, questions, ideas?"

Marnie (county mental health worker): "Boy, we've got a lot of concerning convergence. Frequent UTIs, similar problematic sexual behavior at school and church, dad with a history of sexual misconduct. At best, we've got a girl with frequent UTIs that may be 'checking pooties' because she'd had a lot of medical intervention with regard to her genitals. Worst case . . . well, I think we all know what the worst case is."

Henry: "Well put. We'll let law enforcement and DHS do their jobs with regard to protecting Jennifer and investigating any wrongdoing. But clearly there is a need for intervention here in the interest of protecting the community and attempting to get in the way of Jennifer's problematic sexual behavior. Thoughts?"

Michelle (parole officer): "First, I think we need to get mom involved in this situation. I'm curious what she knows about Rick and about what is going on at school. There may be a great deal we can learn from her. Also, I think we need to put the family on notice. Make sure they understand the need for supervision, and make sure that they understand it is their job to inform their church about increasing supervision. They need to get that if Jennifer harms someone on their watch, it's their responsibility. Again, obviously, if dad is a part of the problem, we can't trust him to be working to protect Jennifer."

Henry: "That's a very good point about the mom. Let's talk about how to bring her in" (discussion continues).

Becky (SRO): "I just got a call from the officer we sent to Rick's house. Turns out mom is home. Our officer just put her in the know about Rick. Officer's impression is that mom had no idea. She's doesn't appear very high functioning, however, so she's likely going to need some support in working through this. Mom asked Rick to leave and our officer is staying at the house until he packs up and goes. Of course, you know how these things work. Mom doesn't have support, so she's going to need some help so she doesn't lose her job."

Reba (DHS): "I wonder if Developmental Disabilities is involved. I can put a call into them today. See if we can get some wraparound for the mom while we sort all this out."

Kurt (Child Sexual Abuse Assessment liaison): "Has the officer spoken to the children?"

Becky: "It doesn't appear so. I think he's waiting for Rick to leave."

Kurt: "I could send someone from our office over if you think that might help."

Becky: "Great. I'll let our officer know to expect someone."

Henry: "Sounds like things are under control. Are there other ideas for this case?" (Discussion continues).

Henry: "Okay. Miguel, I know we talked about a lot of things today. Do you have any questions about the team's recommendations?"

Miguel: "No. I wrote everything down."

Henry: "Great. I'll get the summary to you tomorrow afternoon. Please don't hesitate to contact me if you or your administrator have questions before then. Given how hot this case is right now, I'd recommend that we review it weekly until the situation is stabilized. What does the team think? Looks like we're in agreement. Okay. Let's see what else we have for today. The Bobby Johnson case from three weeks ago. I got an update from the school counselor today that I can share with the group. Steve, I have it written here that you were going to update us as to the status of this case and the pending charges."

Steve (DA's office): "Yep. Got that right here. Looks like . . ." (update continues)

So, there you have it: full case, start to finish. From here, the team will continue to review Jennifer's case until the team decides that the situation is stabilized, at which point they might decide to review it on a monthly, bimonthly, or yearly basis, or to examine the case at Jennifer's next school transition (say from elementary school to middle school), depending upon the need.

As illustrated by this case, it's not important that everything be resolved at the Level 2. You don't need to determine Rick's guilt or innocence. You don't need to make sure that Jennifer is receiving treatment. And you don't need to contact the church to put them on notice.

Your job, as a team, is to connect the dots among the community partners and provide consultation to the school district regarding how to keep students and staff safe while managing the liability of educating a child with problematic sexual behavior.

SALEM KEIZER SCHOOL DISTRICT
SEXUAL INCIDENT RESPONSE SYSTEM
~ LEVEL 1 PROTOCOL ~

(EDITION 2011)

LEVEL 1 OUTCOME
(To be completed at the end of the Level 1 Investigation)

Disposition		Date	Responsible Party
☒	Referred to Law Enforcement	10/5/11	Becky (SRO)
☐	Dismissed		
☒	Developed Supervision Plan	10/6/11	Clinton
☒	Referred to Level 2	10/6/11	Miguel
☐	Other		

Notes: _____

_____

_____

_____

- This system is designed to examine sexual incidents that include concerning/inappropriate sexual behavior. It is not designed for use with students who are suicidal, engaging in threatening/violent behavior or who are setting fires, unless they are doing so as part of a sexual act. (If a suicide screening, threat assessment screening or fire-setting screening is needed, please consult the Salem-Keizer counseling website or call support services at 503.399-3101).

- Consult the flow chart below to determine the course of screening. If a Level 1 Incident Assessment is indicated, proceed with the attached Protocol and step-by-step instructions.

SALEM•KEIZER
PUBLIC SCHOOLS

1

```
   ┌─────────────┐
   │   Sexual    │
   │  Incident   │
   └─────────────┘
```

UPON DISCOVERY OF THE INCIDENT, THE SCHOOL RESOURCE OFFICER SHOULD BE INFORMED. IF THE EVENT IS FOUND TO BE ILLEGAL, REPORT TO LEVEL OFFICES, AND FOLLOW DISTRICT PROTOCOL GUIDELINES.

**Level 1 to be considered by
Administrator & Counselor**

**Guidelines for consideration of
Level 1 (any of the following):**

1. Sexual incident occurs at school.
2. School staff is informed about concerning sexual behavior occurring in school or community.
3. Sexual behavior is causing disruption to school activity.
4. There is a history of sexually inappropriate behavior.
5. Staff, parent, or students perceive the sexual incident as unusual, odd, or inappropriate.
6. Administrator is unable to assert that the concern is unfounded.

Unfounded Concern

Level 1 Protocol completed by Site Team

Steps 1-3:
Demographics and screening.

Step 4:
Use supervision strategies to address concerns. Determine if Level 2 is needed by using suggested criteria.

Step 5: (After completing Level 1) if Level 2 is needed call Wilson Kenney at (503) 689-5709 to schedule.

Step 6:
Sign and Fax a copy of the Level 1 AND incident report to Security Department and appropriate Level Office.

- IMPORTANT -
Maintain two copies of the Level 1: One in a letter-size manila envelope marked "Confidential" placed in the student's regular academic or cumulative file and a second copy in a working file in the administrator's (case manager's) office. Then update SASI to note the presence of a Confidential Record.

SALEM•KEIZER
PUBLIC SCHOOLS

2

**THIS PROTOCOL IS ONLY TO BE USED BY STAFF WHO HAVE BEEN TRAINED
THROUGH THE LEVEL 1 SCREENING PROCESS. READ AT THE START OF EVERY LEVEL 1 MEETING.**
*The results of this survey do not predict or diagnose sexual deviance, nor are they designed to assess an individual's or group's
risk of harm to others. This survey is not a checklist that can be quantified. It is a guide designed to assist Level 1 teams in
making a determination regarding whether the sexual incident in question is normative or non-normative and to assist the school
staff in the development of a management plan. This guide is not intended to serve as an investigation of potential danger and
should not be employed for the purpose of identifying circumstances and variables that may increase risk for potential sexual
misconduct. Furthermore as additional information about a sexual incident is revealed, so may perceptions about the seriousness
of the incident change. If you are reviewing this survey at a date after the assessment completion, do so while being mindful of
supervision, intervention, and the passage of time.*

Complete the following survey through the Site Team Investigation using the noted step-by-step instructions.
The Site Team is composed of the following:

- Administrator (Discipline AP or Principal)
- Counselor
- School Resource Officer (as appropriate)
- Educators or other people who know the student / students

- Parents, if time and circumstances allow / Case Manager if adjudicated or ward of the Court. If parents are unable to attend, complete the Parent Questionnaire through interview.
- Campus Monitor if possible.

Many cases can be managed through a Level 1 Screening with appropriate interventions. The screening usually takes from 20 to 45 minutes and is a way of documenting concerns and management strategies. It is also a way to determine if there is a need to request a more extensive Level 2 Assessment by staff that specializes in Sexual Misconduct investigation (Step 4). If consultation is needed regarding the Level 1 or Level 2 process, please call or email Dr. Wilson Kenney at Student Services (503) 399-3101 or cell (503) 689-5709.

LEVEL 1 SCREENING

STEP 1: MAKE SURE ALL STUDENTS / STAFF ARE SAFE

☐ If necessary take appropriate precautions such as detaining the student and restricting access to coats, backpacks, lockers, etc.

**IF *IMMINENT* DANGER EXISTS CALL LAW ENFORCEMENT, LEVEL OFFICE,
AND FOLLOW THE DISTRICT SAFETY GUIDELINES.**

☐ Notification to parent / guardian of identified targeted student(s) as outlined in district policy.

STEP 2: COMPLETE THE FOLLOWING INFORMATION:

☒ The parent / guardian has been notified that this screening is being done.
☐ The parent / guardian **has not** been notified of this meeting because: _____

☐ Parent questionnaire completed if parent cannot attend (see Sexual Incident Response System Guide).
☐ Parents discouraged from participating by legal counsel.

SCHOOL: Random Elem. SCHOOL PHONE #: 555-1212 TODAY'S DATE: 10/6/11

ADMINISTRATOR / CASE MANAGER: Clinton Doe   DATE OF INCIDENT: 10/5/11

STUDENT NAME: Jennifer Blank STUDENT #: 1234 DOB: 8/11/02 AGE: 9 GRADE: 3

☒ COPY OF **DISTRICT INCIDENT REPORT** IS ATTACHED.

SALEM•KEIZER
PUBLIC SCHOOLS

3

STEP 3: SCREENING – DISCUSS, INVESTIGATE, AND DOCUMENT

Each question is a prompt for exploration of the nature of the sexual incident. Please note concerns by each item or under other concerns **Review the questions below as an outline for a guided conversation investigating the nature of the sexual incident in question.**

Was a report filed with SRO? ☐ No ☒ Yes
☐ Not applicable (historical incident / previous police contact / no current legal concern)

Was event determined to be illegal by the SRO investigation? ☒ No ☐ Yes ☐ Not applicable

Describe details of sexual incident: Jennifer was discovered by Ms. Takahashi in the girls room attempting to digitally penetrate the vagina of a female classroom peer.

PEER TO PEER

1. Are the individuals involved in the sexual incident roughly equivalent in regard to development, cognitive capacity, physical capacity, emotional functioning and coping skills?
☐ No ☒ Yes, if no describe: Unclear. It may be the case that the other student is somewhat cognitively lower.

Note: if individuals differ in regard to age, development or cognitive capacity by three or more years, or if one or more of the individuals involved in the sexual incident are physically incapacitated, the incident in question may represent a concerning power imbalance that warrants further scrutiny.
Consider Supervision Strategies (page 10-11): 18, 20, 50, 52

HISTORICAL DATA
(Gathered via SRO investigation and File Review)

2. Is there a known history of previous sexually inappropriate behavior?
☒ No ☐ Yes, if yes describe: _____
Note: Previous sexually inappropriate behavior suggests that a pattern of maladaptive sexual behavior may be present.

3. Has the student involved in the sexual incident been previously censured, disciplined, or placed on a behavior/safety plan for sexually inappropriate behavior? ☒ No ☐ Yes, if yes describe: ____

Note: Continuing sexually inappropriate behavior in response to censure may suggest a more serious concern regarding sexual misconduct that may warrant closer scrutiny

4. Is there any evidence that the student has been exposed to inappropriate sexual content or behavior?
☒ No ☐ Yes, if yes describe: _____
Note: Research suggests that developmentally premature or inappropriate exposure may play a role in the development of concerning sexual behavior.
Consider Supervision Strategies (page 10-11): 18, 20, 38, 40, 43, 44, 50, 52, 58

SALEM•KEIZER
PUBLIC SCHOOLS

INCIDENT DETAILS

5. Do all parties involved in the sexual incident (when spoken to separately) agree upon the details of the incident?

☒No ☐ Yes, if no describe: Jennifer reports she was helping the girl. The girl claims Jennifer said she was "checking her pootie."

Note: disagreement may reflect dishonesty and the need of one of the members to conceal the degree to which they instigated the sexual incident or attempted to hide its discovery.

6. Were coercion, violence, threats, force, manipulation, gifts, and/or privileges used by one or more parties as a strategy to facilitate compliance with the sexual incident or maintain secrecy?

☒ No ☐ Yes, if yes describe: _____

Note: coercion indicates that at least one of the parties involved in the sexual incident put undue pressure on at least one of the other parties, suggesting that further scrutiny is warranted. Pay particularly close attention to any attempt/effort made by any party to maintain secrecy regarding the incident as this speaks to the degree to which the individual had knowledge that the sexual incident was inappropriate.
Consider Supervision Strategies (page 10-11): 6, 40, 43, 49, 50, 51, 52

7. Was the sexual behavior consistent with developmentally normative/common sexual conduct?

☒No ☐ Yes, if no describe: Unusual for a female Jennifer's age to have interest in vaginally penetrating a peer.

Note: developmentally atypical sexual behavior may suggest pathological sexual development that warrants further scrutiny.
Consider Supervision Strategies (page 10-11): 40, 43, 50, 52, 58

8. Did the sexual incident cause physical or emotional pain or discomfort to any of the involved parties?

☒No ☐ Yes, if yes describe: _____

Note: sexual behavior that causes emotional, physical pain and/or psychological distress to others suggests that the event in question was harmful and should be examined with further scrutiny.
Consider Supervision Strategies (page 10-11): 40, 50, 52

9. What does the student indicate was the motive for the sexual behavior (how do they explain it)?

Describe: Unclear. She claimed to the girl she was "checking her pootie".

Note: Poor insight, deceptiveness, lack of empathy and minimization may suggest the need for intervention is higher than when these areas are not compromised.
Consider Supervision Strategies (page 10-11): 40, 50, 52

10. Was there an obvious imbalance in power (difference in physical strength or access to opportunity/resources) among the individuals involved in the sexual incident?
☒ No ☐ Yes, if yes describe: _____

Note: an imbalance of power may suggest that coercion played a role in the sexual incident.
Consider Supervision Strategies (page 10-11): 6, 40, 43, 49, 50, 51, 52

11. Was a weapon present during the sexual incident?
☒ No ☐ Yes, if yes describe: _____

Note: a weapon refers to any object that may be used to threaten physical or emotional safety (i.e. not limited to conventional weapons such as knives or firearms). The mere presence of a weapon, whether employed in a threatening manner or not, may suggest that coercion was employed.
Consider Supervision Strategies (page 10-11): 6, 40, 43, 49, 50, 51, 52

12. Did grooming occur in the context of the sexual incident (refer to the Grooming Behaviors?
☒ No ☐ Yes, if yes describe: _____

Note: grooming suggests that strong sexual intent and manipulation played a role in the sexual incident which may require further scrutiny.
Consider Supervision Strategies (page 10-11): 40, 50, 52

13. Did staff, parents or others voice a strong visceral response regarding the sexual incident?
☐ No ☒ Yes, if yes describe: Staff are concerned about the
event and how the parent responded.
Note: a strong visceral response suggests that individuals have a serious concern that is difficult to verbalize. Further scrutiny of the incident is recommended.

OTHER CONCERNS

Enuretic/Encopretic? ☐ No ☐ Yes Past / Present *Consider Supervision Strategies:40, 49*	**Impulsive?** ☐ No ☐ Yes *Consider Supervision Strategies: 13, 15*	
Harms Animals? ☐ No ☐ Yes Past / Present *Consider Supervision Strategies:40, 49*	**Opportunistically Vigilant?** ☐ No ☒ Yes *Consider Supervision Strategies :15, 17, 20, 21,*	
Planful? ☐ No ☐ Yes *Consider Supervision Strategies:30, 40, 49*		

Threatening Behavior

Suicidal Ideation? ☐ No ☐ Yes Past / Present *Consider Supervision Strategies: 4, 5, 40, 49*	☐ Refer for Suicide Risk Assessment
Targeted Threat? ☐ No ☐ Yes Past / Present *Consider Supervision Strategies:6, 40, 49*	☐ Refer for Student Threat Assessment
Firesetting? ☐ No ☐ Yes Past / Present *Consider Supervision Strategies: 7, 40, 49*	☐ Refer for Firesetting Assessment

SALEM•KEIZER
PUBLIC SCHOOLS

Other Concerns (DHS involvement, multiple foster placements, mental health concerns, health concerns, important historical factors, exposure to abuse/neglect, current mood, sleep routine, appetite, medication, familial history of sexual misconduct, etc.):

Family is new to the district. Little known about supports or complicating factors. Some indication that the family attends church.

Based upon the aforementioned information:
Circle the nature of the sexual incident of concern
Sexual Behavior Continuum (Consider AGE, FORCE and CONTEXT as a factor)

Lower Concern ◄————————————————————————► Higher Concern

- Flirting/Sexual Harassment
- Public kissing/hugging
- Peeping
- Sexual talk/drawing/gesturing
- Rubbing pubic area against object
- Public masturbation
- Exposing sexual parts
- Over the clothes sexual touching
- Rubbing pubic area against person
- Under the clothes non-penetrative sexual touching
- Penetrative sexual touching
- Penetrative sex

CONSIDER REQUESTING A <u>LEVEL 2 SEXUAL INCIDENT RESPONSE</u> IF:

1. The sexual incident appears non-normative and/or severe with regard to intensity, **and / or**
2. You have clear concerns but are unable to confidently answer questions on this protocol, **and / or**
3. You have confidently answered the questions on this protocol and have safety concerns that are beyond your Site Team's ability to supervise and secure within the building, **and / or**
4. You have exhausted your building resources and would like to explore community support to assist you with supervision. **and/or**

See Step 5 for Level 2 Sexual Incident Response referral process.

SALEM•KEIZER
PUBLIC SCHOOLS

7

LEVEL 1 OUTCOME
(To be completed at the end of the Level 1 Investigation)

Disposition	Date	Responsible Party
☒ Refer to Law Enforcement	10/5/11	Becky (SRO)
☐ Dismiss		
☒ Develop Supervision Plan	10/6/11	Clinton
☒ Refer to Level 2	10/6/11	Miguel

Notification & Release	Date	Responsible Party
☐ DHS		
☐ Law Enforcement		
☐ Private Therapist		
☐ Liberty House		
☐ Juvenile Justice		

Notes: _Parent unwilling to sign._
–

_____

–

Participants:

_____
Administrator   **Other:**

_____
Counselor   **Other:**

_____
SRO   **Other:**

SALEM·KEIZER
PUBLIC SCHOOLS

STEP 4: DEVELOP A SUPERVISION PLAN TO ADDRESS CONCERNS
(Including aggravating factors) IDENTIFIED THROUGH STEP 3.

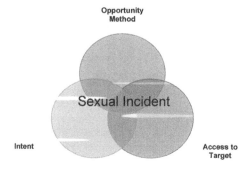

Opportunity
Method

Sexual Incident

Intent   Access to
Target

Sexual Incidents occur at the intersection of Opportunity, Access and Intent.
In supervision planning, one should be mindful of the degree to which our strategies limit
Access and Opportunity, and consider the nature of the student's Intent.

Perceived Intent:
- ☒ Engage in concerning sexual behavior
- ☐ Unknown
- ☐ Other (Specify):_____

Target (mark all that apply):
- ☐ Younger children (specify age):_____
- ☒ Peers
- ☐ Compromised Peers (specify):_____
- ☐ Adults

- ☐ Males
- ☒ Females
- ☐ Other:_____

Opportunities (mark all that apply):
- ☐ Transitions/Lining-up
- ☐ Recess/Lunch/Assemblies
- ☒ Bathroom
- ☐ Technology use
- ☐ Bus
- ☐ Aftercare

- ☐ Classroom
- ☐ Walking Home
- ☐ Community
- ☐ Home
- ☐ Other:_____

SALEM•KEIZER
PUBLIC SCHOOLS

STEP 4 *Continued*

RECOMMENDED INTERVENTIONS (CHECK ☒ IF IMPLEMENTED):
Bolded Items are typically included in most supervision plans

Individual Options:
1. ☐ Intended victim warned – parent/guardian notified (see Notification form)
2. ☐ Protective Response initiated by Security Department
3. ☒ **Individual Accountability Plan**
   Detail Expectations of Plan (e.g. **Hands to work, No sexual talk, etc.**): Inform Jennifer of her supervision plan. Make clear no sexual touching at school.
4. ☐ Suicide Assessment initiated on _____ (use District Suicide Protocol)
   _{date}
5. ☐ No harm contract
6. ☐ Threat Assessment initiated on _____ (use District Threat Assessment Protocol)
   _{date}
7. ☐ Firesetter Assessment initiated on _____ (use District Firesetter Assessment Protocol)
   _{date}
8. ☐ Other: _____

School Options:
9. ☐ Bus Supervision, Specify:_____
10. ☐ Student Escorted from Transport to School Office, and from Classroom to Transport by:_____
11. ☐ Student Escorted from School Office to Classroom and back by Adult, Specify:_____
12. ☒ **Line-of-Sight Supervision (Zone)**
13. ☐ Arms-Reach Supervision (One-on-one)
14. ☐ Supervised Lunch/Breaks/Recess/Assembly
15. ☐ Special Classroom Seating Assignment (to increase supervision)
16. ☐ No After-School Activities
17. ☐ Supervised After-School Activities (Specify in Safety Plan)
18. ☐ Academic Restrictions (e.g. not involved in childcare courses, mentoring younger students, technology)
   Specify:_____
19. ☐ No Access to Technology
20. ☐ Supervised Access to Technology
21. ☒ Bathroom Plan, Specify: Use staff restroom.
22. ☐ Review educational plan
23. ☐ Social Work Services
24. ☐ Travel card and time accountability
25. ☐ Social skills building programs
26. ☐ Increase supervision in following settings in the following ways: _____
27. ☐ Modifications of daily schedule ☐ Late arrival / early dismissal
28. ☒ **Alert staff on need-to-know basis, Specify staff:**
   ☐ All supervisory staff ☐ Teacher only ☒ Teacher and I.A.'s only ☒ SRO ☒ Office staff
   Staff member responsible for alerting staff and teachers: Clinton Doe
29. ☐ Random Check of backpack, locker, pocket, purse, etc. by:
   ☐ Administrator ☐ CDS / Counselor ☐ SRO ☐ Office staff ☐ Other_____
30. ☐ Assign identified staff to build trusting relationship through check-in or mentorship:
   ☐ Administrator ☐ Mentor ☐ CDS/ Counselor ☐ School Resource Officer ☐ Teacher ☐ Other: _____
31. ☐ Other interventions or supervision strategies that will likely decrease the possibility of a future sexual incident
   Describe: _____

SALEM•KEIZER
PUBLIC SCHOOLS

STEP 4 *Continued*

(NOTE: If student is on IEP/504 plan, any change in placement or Special Ed services must be done through Special Education Team process or 504 team process.)

32. ☐ Referral to appropriate school team to consider alternative placement
33. ☐ Home supervision pending further assessment
34. ☐ Increased supervision in the following settings: _____
35. ☐ Referral to appropriate Special Ed. Team to consider Psycho Educational Evaluation / Special Education Assessment or Behavior Team Referral. **(NOTE: Must be done through Special Education Team Process.)**

☐ Other: _____
_____

Family / Home Options:

Guardians encouraged to:
36. ☐ No Access to Technology
37. ☐ Supervised Access to Technology
38. ☐ Line-of-Sight Supervision
39. ☐ Safety Proof home
40. ☐ Review & pursue crisis/mental health services
41. ☒ **Provide detailed information regarding safety concerns to care providers when leaving child in care of others**
42. ☐ Increase supervision (specify): _____
_____

43. ☐ Guardian discouraged from allowing sleepovers
44. ☐ Guardian provided list of treatment providers
45. ☐ **Guardian provided list of concerning / grooming behaviors**
46. ☒ **Guardian discouraged from allowing contact between students involved in sexual incident**
47. ☐ Other: _____
_____

Clinton to provide information to family.

Encouraged Community Options:

_____ encouraged to pursue:
(community organization)
48. ☐ Referral to YST
49. ☐ Mental Health evaluation
50. ☐ Psychosexual evaluation
51. ☐ Anger management programs
52. ☐ Sexual Misconduct / Interpersonal Boundaries programs
53. ☐ Alcohol / Drug evaluation

54. ☐ Parenting Programs
55. ☐ Mentoring programs
56. ☐ Notify Probation / Parole officer
57. ☐ Faith Based Community Programs
58. ☐ Liberty House
59. ☐ Mid-Valley Women's Crisis Center

Other Options: _____
_____
_____
_____

Review:
☒ Administrator will review the status of this plan and revise as needed on: ___11/11/11___
                                                                                (date)

SALEM•KEIZER
PUBLIC SCHOOLS

STEP 5: After completion of the Level 1 Screening, and if the Site Team has determined that a Level 2 Meeting is needed,

Immediately contact **Wilson Kenney** at **(503) 689-5709** to begin the process and

Fax a copy of the Level 1 to **Rhonda Stueve** at **(503) 375-7815**.

Please provide Dispatch with the information requested below so a complete Level 2 team can be assembled in a timely manner.

If a Level 2 Response is not requested, move to Step 6 to complete the protocol.

NOTE:

While awaiting the Level 2 Response, use the student supervision plan (Step 4) to manage the situation and document interim steps taken by Site Team.

INFORMATION NEEDED FOR DISPATCHING A LEVEL 2

1. Is student adjudicated? ☐ Yes ☒ No
   If yes – Name of Probation Officer _____ Phone #:_____

2. A Ward of the Court or other supervision? ☐ Yes ☒ No
   If yes – Name of Caseworker _____ Phone#: _____

3. Other agencies or individuals involved with the student (therapists, doctors, etc.) that should be included with the parent's permission? ☐ Yes ☐ No
   If yes, is there signed consent for exchange of information? ☐ Yes ☒ No
   If yes, please list agencies and individuals: _____ Phone: _____
   _____ Phone: _____
   _____ Phone: _____

4. Special Ed. Or 504 involvement, disability codes and current placement? ☒ Yes ☐ No
   If yes, details: _Speech and language._

5. Is student in self-contained classroom? ☐ Yes ☒ No

6. Was parent or guardian present at Level 1 survey: ☒ Yes ☐ No

7. Are parents supportive, constructive and available to attend Level 2? ☐ Yes ☒ No
   If yes, what is their contact information: Home Phone:_____Cell Phone:_____

8. Other information Level 2 team will need for assessment: _Little known about the family. Father walked out of Level 1._

SALEM•KEIZER
PUBLIC SCHOOLS

STEP 6:
Sign, send, file and begin supervision as planned.

1. Sign the Protocol
2. Fax a copy of the Level 1 Protocol to Rhonda Stueve (503) 375-7815

3. Fax a copy of the Level 1 Protocol to the *Appropriate* Level Office:
   Elementary Education: (503) 375-7804
   Secondary Education (503) 375-7817

4. Maintain two copies of the Level 1.
   One in a letter-size manila envelope marked "Confidential Record" placed in the student's regular academic or cumulative file and *a second* copy in a working file in the Administrator's (case manager's) office.

5. Then update SASI to note the presence of a Confidential Record.

Team Signatures:

Administrator, Plan Supervisor	Date	Counselor	Date
School Resource Officer	Date	Other	Date
Parent	Date	Other	Date
Other	Date	Other	Date
Other	Date	Other	Date

Developed by Wilson Kenney, Ph.D. at Salem-Keizer Public Schools using the following information: VanDreal, Salem-Keizer School District Threat Assessment Response System; Friedrich, Fisher, Broughton, Houston and Shafran; Barbaree and Marshall, The Juvenile Sex Offender; Normative Sexual Behavior in Children: A Contemporary Sample; NCSBY Fact Sheet.; Kaeser, Towards a Better Understanding of Children's Sexual Behavior; Elliot, Grooming; Stewart, Victim Grooming: Protect your Child from Sexual Predators; Anderson, Continuum of Sexual Behavior; Pynchon and Borum, Assessing Threats of Targeted Group Violence: Contributions from Social Psychology; Reddy, Borum, Berlun, Vossekuil, Fein, and Modzeleski, Evaluating Risk for Targeted Violence in Schools: Comparing Risk Assessment, Threat Assessment, and Other Approaches; O'Toole, The School Shooter: A Threat Assessment Perspective; Fein, Vossekuil and Holden, Threat Assessment: An Approach to Prevent Targeted Violence; Meloy, Violence Risk and Threat Assessment, Specialized Training Services Publication; De Becker, The Gift of Fear; Vossekuil, Pollack, Bourne, Modzekski, Reddy, and Fein, Threat Assessment in Schools, A Guide to Managing Threatening Situations and to Creating Safe School Climates.

SALEM·KEIZER
PUBLIC SCHOOLS

SEXUAL INCIDENT RESPONSE AND MANAGEMENT SYSTEM
Sexual Incident Inquiry
~ Level 2~

> This protocol was developed by Wilson Kenney, School Psychologist, Salem-Keizer School District. It is a structured outline to be used only by professionals trained in SIRC inquiry, mental health/behavioral assessment, and psychoeducational assessment.

Student Name(s): <u>Jennifer Blank</u> Age: <u>9</u> Grade: <u>3</u> Student Number(s): <u>1234</u> DOB: <u>8/11/02</u>

Today's Date: <u>10/7/11</u> School: <u>Random Elem</u>. Administrative Case Manager: <u>Clinton Doe.</u>

Description of the Incident: <u>Jennifer was discovered digitally penetrating the vagina of a female peer while in the restroom. Jennifer denied the touching. The female peer reported Jennifer claimed she needed to "check her pootie."</u>

- ☐ 504 ☒ Spec. Ed ☐ Regular Ed ☐ Adjudication ☐ Ward of State/Court ☐ Foster Care

- Testing information if available:

  Speech and language. No testing available.

- Disciplinary action taken:

  Admin spoke with student about incident.

- Safety planning put in place by school:

  Bathroom plan.
  Line of sight supervision.

SITUATION OR INCIDENT FACTORS:

Targets of Concern

☐ Younger children (specify age):_____
☒ Peers
☑ Compromised Peers
(specify):_____
☐ Adults

☐ Males
☒ Females
☐ Other:_____

4/1/10

SALEM·KEIZER
PUBLIC SCHOOLS

Sexual Behavior Continuum
Consider AGE, FORCE and CONTEXT as a factor

←──→

Flirting/Sexual Harassment	Public kissing/hugging	Peeping	Sexual talk/drawing/gesturing	Frotteurism toward an object	Public masturbation	Exposing sexual parts	Over the clothes sexual touching	Frotteurism toward a person	Under the clothes non-penetrative sexual touching	Penetrative sexual touching	Penetrative sex

Details suggesting that the incident was concerning:

- ☒ Significant difference (>3 years) in regard to:
  - ☐ Age
  - ☒ Cognitive development – Possible
  - ☒ Emotional development (coping skills, behavior)
  - ☐ Physical capacity
- ☐ History of sexually inappropriate bx
- ☐ Previously censured for sexually inappropriate bx
- ☒ Disagreement regarding details of incident
- ☐ Evidence of grooming
- ☒ Strong visceral response among staff/parents
- ☐ Confusion/Discomfort among involved parties

- ☐ Attempts at gaining compliance/secrecy:
  - ☐ Coercion
  - ☐ Violence (or threat of violence)
  - ☐ Force
  - ☐ Manipulation
  - ☐ Gifts/Privileges
- ☒ Developmentally non-normative incident
- ☐ Incident caused physical/emotional pain
- ☐ Confusion about appropriateness of incident
- ☐ Imbalance of power
- ☐ Weapon was present

Suggested nature of the of the incident/concern:

Normative		Non-normative	

←──X──→

Normative Affection Playful Flirting	Sexually Normative but Mutually Inappropriate Sexual Behavior	Sexually Aggressive & Sexually Non-normative Behavior	Illegal Sexual Behavior

- Preparation/grooming related behavior?

  None noted

4/1/10

- Other students / people involved (supporting / allowing acting out, ideation, planning)?

    Student Name(s):_____Age:___Grade: _____ (Level 1 or Level 2 assessment complete? Y/N)

    _____ ___ _____ (Level 1 or Level 2 assessment complete? Y/N)

    _____ ___ _____ (Level 1 or Level 2 assessment complete? Y/N)

- Motive?

    Unclear. Jennifer denies the event.

- Circumstances that might increase risk for sexual misconduct:

- Inhibitors and protective factors (stable living situation, student manages anger well, student has support system, student appears concerned about managing sexual behavior, student recognizes need for support, student recognizes risk factors, student demonstrates willingness to follow safety plan):

    Unclear. Father walked out of Level 1. Family attends church ... may be a protective factor but also domain in which further concerning sexual behavior could occur.

Situation/Incident factor concerns are:

☐ **Unremarkable / low**   ☐ **Decreasing**   ☒ **Ongoing**   ☐ **Escalating**

SALEM•KEIZER
PUBLIC SCHOOLS

SCHOOL FACTORS

- Academics:

  Below average in reading and math. Some concern about cognitive. May recommend testing once previous testing can be reviewed.
- Attendance:

  Generally good.

- Attachment to school:

  Unclear.

- Behavioral history:

  None noted.

- Discipline history:

- Educational goals or plan:

  IEP attached.

- Other School Concerns:

School factor concerns are:
☐ **Unremarkable / low**   ☐ **Decreasing**   ☐ **Ongoing**   ☐ **Escalating**

SOCIAL FACTORS

- Relationships with non-family adults (teachers, community leaders, church, clubs, etc.):

  New student. Not yet connected.

- Interpersonal history at school, home and community (real or perceived):

  Unclear.

- Social status

  Not yet part of social milieu. Not yet connected to peers.

- Peer group (culture, subculture, clique or marginalized clique).

- Role within peer group

- Peers, culture or community endorse unhealthy sexual attitudes?

- Community support level:

Social factor concerns are:
☐ **Unremarkable / low**   ☐ **Decreasing**   ☒ **Ongoing**   ☐ **Escalating**

SALEM•KEIZER
PUBLIC SCHOOLS

4/1/10

PERSONAL FACTORS

- Pattern of behavior: UNKNOWN

- Personally views sexual behavior as acceptable and normative?

- Emotional coping skills and reserves

- Attitude
  ☐ self as superior   ☐ has healthy view of personal strengths and weaknesses
  ☐ sees self as a victim   ☐ sees self as a failure
  ☐ entitled   ☐ sees self as inferior, broken or weak
  ☐ criminal   ☐ other:_____
  ☐ narcissistic

- Stress level (real or perceived):

- Concerns
  ☐ awareness of dysfunctional or troubled situation and wants to change
  ☐ has awareness but lacks concern or doesn't care
  ☐ is unaware of dysfunctional or troubled situation

- Trust level:

Sexual Behavior/Attitudes:

- Previously adjudicated for sexual misconduct
  ☐ >2 previous victims of sexual abuse   ☐ previous offense/s involved violence
  ☐ previous offense/s suggests planning   ☐ offended same victim >1
  ☐ previous offense/s involved coercion   ☐ attempt to hide previous sexual misconduct
  ☐ penetrative sexual act
  Previous victim/s:
  ☐ male only   ☐ female only   ☐ both   ☐ > 3 year age difference developmentally
  ☐ interfamilial   ☐ extrafamilial   ☐ stranger

- Previously attended treatment for sexual misconduct
  ☐ Successfully completed   ☐ Failed to complete   ☐ Maximum benefit

- Past treatment/intervention accessibility and response
  ☐ accessible   ☐ guarded   ☐ poor response   ☐ resistive   ☐ hostile

4/1/10

FAMILY DYNAMIC FACTORS

- Resides with:

  Father, mother, and younger sister.

- Siblings?

  1 younger

- Custody?

  Parents appear to have custody.

- Familial history of: *– unclear*
  - ☐ Domestic Violence   ☐ Neglect   ☐ Criminal activity
  - ☐ Mental illness   ☐ Substance abuse   ☐ Previous sanctions for sexual misconduct
  - ☐ Abuse

- Parents /guardians support level:

  Low SES … may benefit from support / outreach

- Family dynamic and relationships (parental, sibling):

  Father stays at home with girls. Mother works.

- Parents and or family views regarding sexual behavior?

  Conservative

- Lack of supervision within the household?

  unclear – father claims supervision is high.

- Family is interested in seeking treatment/help for student?

  Father appears hostile to Level I process.

- Family is concerned about students sexual behavior?

  unclear

- Poor parental control and/or few limits on behavior?

  unclear

- Computer access within home? Supervised computer access?

  unclear

- Extended family support level:

  unclear

Family Dynamic factor concerns are:
☐ Unremarkable / low   ☐ Decreasing   ☒ Ongoing   ☐ Escalating

4/1/10

SALEM•KEIZER
PUBLIC SCHOOLS

SEXUAL INCIDENT RESPONSE AND MANAGEMENT SYSTEM
Summary of Level 2 Inquiry

Today's Date: 10/8/11   Date of Incident: 10/5/11   School: Random Elem.

Student Name(s): Jennifer Blank   Student Number(s): 1234

Name of Other Students if Involved: _____

_____

DOB: 8/11/02 Age: 9 Grade: 3 Administrative Case Manager: Clinton

> This summary was generated through the efforts of the sexual incident response system (a set of protocols used by members of the Sexual Incident Response Committee referred to as "SIRC"). The summary: 1) identifies concerns that arose during the case investigation, 2) communicates the case disposition (i.e. interventions, supervision/safety planning, and risk mitigation strategies that were recommended) and 3) identifies the factors that suggest additional risk mitigation planning is warranted. It should be noted that this summary is not a psychosexual report or a prediction of future risk for sexual misconduct, nor is it a foolproof method of assessing an individual's short or long-term risk of harming others sexually. Since it is an examination of current circumstances (and as these circumstances change, so too does the disposition), please review the contents while being mindful of supervision, intervention and the passage of time. For information regarding the Level 1 or Level 2 threat assessment process or the contents of this report, please contact SIRC as represented by J. Wilson Kenney, Salem-Keizer School District (503) 399-3101.

SEXUAL INCIDENT RESPONSE COMMITTEE (SIRC)
The Sexual Incident Response Committee or SIRC is comprised of the following: Salem-Keizer School District, Willamette Educational Services District (WESD), Marion County Sheriff's Office, Salem Police Department, Keizer Police Department, Oregon Judicial Department, Marion County Children's Mental Health, Polk County Children's Mental Health, Marion County Juvenile Dept., Polk County Juvenile Dept., Oregon Youth Authority and Oregon Department of Human Services. SIRC is a consultation team that examines concerning sexual incidents that impact education and assists case managers with the application of resources to manage and decrease the possibility of future sexual misconduct, and support students to develop and employ healthy and safe coping strategies.

REFERRAL

This student was referred for Level 2 threat assessment because:

☒ The sexual incident appears non-normative,

☐ Staff have clear concerns but are unable to confidently answer questions on this protocol,

☒ Staff have confidently answered the questions on this protocol and have safety concerns that are beyond the Site Team's ability to supervise and secure within the building,

☐ Staff have exhausted building resources and would like to explore community support to assist with supervision.

☐ Other: _____

SALEM•KEIZER
PUBLIC SCHOOLS

INCIDENT/CONCERN

The following is a description of the incident or concern: Jennifer was discovered digitally penetrating the vagina of a female peer while in the restroom.

Context in which the incident occurred and details of the incident:

Place: Girls bathroom

Structure level:
- ☒ Low
- ☐ Moderate
- ☐ High
- ☐ Any

Social situation: Peers were largely unknown to one another. Not friends.

Target of sexual behavior:
- ☒ Females
- ☐ Males
- ☐ Adults
- ☐ Developmentally equivalent peers
- ☐ Developmentally compromised peers
- ☐ Younger children: _____ age range
- ☐ other: _____

Expression of sexual behavior:
- ☐ Sexual talk / drawings
- ☐ Sexually aggressive posturing
- ☐ Sexual kissing
- ☐ Frotteurism (rubbing genitals against someone/something)
- ☐ Exposing genitals
- ☐ Public masturbation

- ☐ Over the clothes sexual touching of others
- ☒ Under the clothes sexual touching of others
- ☐ Penetrative sex
- ☐ Threatened forcible sex
- ☐ Forced sex
- ☐ other: _____

- ☐ Influenced by peer pressure or gang related:
- ☐ Influenced by drugs and alcohol:
- ☒ Criminal act: SRO sent referral to D.A.

Details suggesting that the incident was concerning:
- ☐ Significant difference (>3 years) in regard to:
  - ☐ Age
  - ☒ Cognitive development – Possible
  - ☐ Emotional development (coping skills, behavior)
  - ☐ Physical capacity
- ☐ History of sexually inappropriate bx
- ☐ Previously censured for sexually inappropriate bx
- ☒ Disagreement regarding details of incident
- ☐ Evidence of grooming
- ☒ Strong visceral response among staff/parents
- ☐ Confusion/Discomfort among involved parties

- ☐ Attempts at gaining compliance/secrecy:
  - ☐ Coercion
  - ☐ Violence (or threat of violence)
  - ☐ Force
  - ☐ Manipulation
  - ☐ Gifts/Privileges
- ☒ Developmentally non-normative incident
- ☐ Incident caused physical/emotional pain
- ☐ Confusion about appropriateness of incident
- ☐ Imbalance of power
- ☐ Weapon was present

INCIDENT/CONCERN:

Sexual Behavior Continuum
Consider AGE, FORCE and CONTEXT as a factor

◄──►

| Flirting/Sexual Harassment | Public kissing/hugging | Peeping | Sexual talk/drawing/gesturing | Frotteurism toward an object | Public masturbation | Exposing sexual parts | Over the clothes sexual touching | Frotteurism toward a person | Under the clothes non-penetrative sexual touching | Penetrative sexual touching | Penetrative sex |

Suggested nature of the of the incident/concern:

Normative	Non-normative

◄──►

| Normative Affection Playful Flirting | Sexually Normative but Mutually Inappropriate Sexual Behavior | Sexually Aggressive & Sexually Non-normative Behavior | Illegal Sexual Behavior |

Recommended response as a function of continuum:

Green: Continue to monitor through normal school protocol

Yellow: In most cases, unless the act is egregious, repetitive in spite of discipline, or developmentally unusual
1. Talk with Students
2. Talk with Parents (and any others involved in the incident)
3. Execute Administrative Discipline
4. Document

Orange: Refer to Level 2 Facilitator and,
1. Talk with Students
2. Talk with Parents
3. Execute Administrative Discipline
4. Document

Red: Contact Police

CASE DISPOSITION & RECOMMENDATIONS

These recommendations were generated through the efforts of the 24-J Sexual Incident Response Committee (SIRC) and are for consideration in the management of sexually concerning incidents and circumstances involving students. SIRC is a consultation team that investigates sexual incidents and assists case managers with the application of resources to manage and decrease the possibility of future sexual misconduct, and support students to develop and employ healthy and safe sexual behavior.

(CHECK ☒ IF RECOMMENDED)

Next Steps:

☒ Case will be staffed by Sexual Incident Response Committee (SIRC). *Review on 10/15/11*
☒ Administrator will request further assessment if risk circumstances escalate. Call: (503)-399-3101.

☒ Continue with Level 1 Student Supervision Plan
☐ Intended victim warned
☐ Parent / Guardian of targeted student notified

Student Options:

☒ Individual Accountability Plan: No harm contract / Student will self manage: Describe: *Student informed of plan.*
☐ Suicide Assessment initiated on _____ (use District Suicide Protocol.)
☐ Student Threat Assessment initiated on _____ (use STAT Protocol.)
☐ Student Firesetter Assessment initiated on _____ (use District Firesetter Protocol.)
☐ Student will identify triggers, agitators and agree to "safe room" or resource of support.
☐ Diversion

School Options:

☐ Protective Response initiated by Security Department
☒ Alert staff and teachers on need-to-know basis
☐ Bus Supervision (Specify in Safety Plan)
☐ Student Escorted from Bus to School Office, and from Classroom to School Bus
☐ Student Escorted to and from School Office by Adult, Specify: _____
☒ Line-of-Sight Supervision
☐ Arms-Reach Supervision
☐ Supervised Lunch/Breaks/Recess/Assembly
☐ Special Classroom Seating Assignment (to increase supervision)
☐ No After-School Activities
☐ Supervised After-School Activities (Specify in Safety Plan)
☐ Academic Restrictions (e.g. not involved in childcare courses, or mentoring younger students)
☐ No Access to Technology
☐ Supervised Access to Technology
☒ Review educational plan
☐ Specialized class / Alternative class or track
☐ Travel card and time accountability
☐ Late arrival / early dismissal
☐ Entry / Exit check with:
☒ Continue to monitor communications and behavior.
☒ Other School option: *Bathroom plan.*

☐ Social skill building programs
☐ Increase supervision in following settings:
☐ Decrease or eliminate pass time or unsupervised time
☐ Daily ☐ Weekly modification of schedule:
☐ Random search of backpack/purse, locker, pockets, etc. by school personnel:
☒ Assign identified staff to build trusting relationship through check-in or mentorship:
    ☐ Administrator ☒ Counselor ☐ Mentor
    ☐ School Resource Officer ☐ Teacher ☐ Other:
☐ Provide means by which student may safely report and discuss thoughts or intentions to harm others and receive appropriate intervention.
☐ Identify and further develop activities, relationships or things of value that inhibit possibility of acting out:
☐ Other interventions or supervision strategies that will directly address the triggers and agitators identified through assessment:
☐ School Counselor intervention including:
☐ Refer to PIRS or other school resource:
☐ Consider placement change (administrative transfer, Interim Alternative Educational Setting (IAES), expulsion, etc. as per district policy. (District may unilaterally remove student to IAES, but IEP team decides actual placement if student is receiving specialized instruction. See gray box below.)
☐ Safety planning at site of attendance (home school; SPED placement; Alternative Ed.; IDT.

SALEM•KEIZER
PUBLIC SCHOOLS

CASE DISPOSITION & RECOMMENDATIONS

☒ Refer to school special education or 504 team to consider evaluation. If student has IEP or 504 plan refer to special education team or 504 team to consider: *Student may require additional testing.*
- ☐ Further evaluation
- ☐ Reviewing goals and placement options
- ☐ Referral to alternative educational placement
- ☐ Increasing supervision in the following setting: _____
- ☐ Home supervision pending further assessment or action.

Family / Home Options:
- ☐ Strategize Safety options / planning
- ☐ Increase supervision
- ☐ No Access to Technology
- ☐ Supervised Access to Technology
- ☒ Line-of-Sight Supervision
- ☐ Locked Bedrooms for Family Members

Community Options:
- ☐ Referral to YST
- ☐ School referred (STAT) mental health valuation
- ☐ Anger management programs
- ☐ Mentoring programs
- ☐ Notify Probation /Parole officer
- ☐ Faith Community Programs
- ☐ Foster Positive Community Activities, interests
- ☐ Refer to Juvenile Family Support Program

Other Options:

- ☐ Parents contacted and will provide following supervision / intervention:
- ☐ Safety proof home
- ☐ Referral for Domestic Violence intervention
- ☐ Parent training classes.
- ☒ Other: *Parents informed of responsibility to inform care providers of threat.*
- ☐ Explore grant money assistance for inhibitors or other needs
- ☐ Referral to substance abuse intervention with:
- ☐ Referral to Mental Health agency for mental health evaluation contact:
- ☐ Review of counseling or therapy options.
- ☐ Juvenile Dept. supervision and release / safety plan
- ☒ Other: *Mother referred to D.V. support.*

Also parents discouraged from having contact with student outside of school and from allowing sleepovers.

FACTORS SUGGESTIVE THAT ADDITIONAL RISK MITIGATION PLANNING MAY BE WARRANTED

Context in which future incidents may be more likely to occur:

Place: Bathroom, unsupervised settings.

Structure level:

☒ Low ☐ Moderate ☐ High ☐ Any

Social situation: Jennifer seems willing

Target of sexual behavior:	Expression of sexual behavior:	

☒ Females
☐ Males
☐ Adults
☐ Developmentally
   equivalent peers
☐ Developmentally
   compromised peers
☐ Younger children: ____
                age range
☐ other:_____
	☐ Sexual talk
	☐ Sexually aggressive
	   posturing
	☐ Sexual kissing
	☐ Frotteurism (rubbing
	   genitals against
	   someone/something)
	☐ Exposing genitals
	☐ Public masturbation
		☐ Over the clothes sexual
		   touching of others
		☒ Under the clothes sexual
		   touching of others
		☐ Penetrative sex
		☐ Threatened forcible sex
		☐ Forced sex
		☐ other:_____

☐ Influenced by peer pressure or gang related:
☐ Influenced by drugs and alcohol:
☐ Criminal act:

Factors which suggest the need for additional consideration

☐ New allegations ☒ Student violates supervision plan ☐ Student's therapist/supervision officer/guardian suggests the need for additional supervision ☐ Student evidences recent escalation in anger or negative affect ☐ Student evidences sudden change in affect/behavior	☐ Student appears to be socially isolating self ☐ Student appears to be actively grooming other students ☐ Student evidencing interpersonal aggression toward others ☐ Recent change in caregiver or living situation ☐ Sudden change in school performance

SUMMARY

If a student's situation changes please call (503) 510-8924 to schedule a review of this case.

Further information regarding this assessment is available by contacting the Case Manager (Administrator) at the student's school, the Liaison Officer assigned to that school or the Sexual Incident Response Committee (as represented by Wilson Kenney at Salem-Keizer School District, Student Services, (503) 399-3101.)

_____

Wilson Kenney, Ph.D.
School Psychologist

Copy of Report to: * Wilson Kenney
                      * School Site Team

SALEM-KEIZER
PUBLIC SCHOOLS

Chapter 9

Title IX

Mary Kane and Liane O'Banion

Title IX of the Education Amendments Act is an often misunderstood, sometimes controversial, and frequently wrongly maligned law that has important bearing on the work of protecting students from sexual harm. It is apparent that the work of SIRC bumps up against Title IX but it's not immediately clear how these elements can and should fit together. The following chapter, which was written by Mary Kane, JD (legal counsel at Portland Public School) and Liane O'Banion, EdD (Title IX director at Portland Public School), provides an excellent example of how the largest district in Oregon elegantly incorporates these two systems in a collaborative fashion.

TITLE IX THROUGH THE YEARS

Title IX of the Education Amendments Act was codified in 1972 by the federal government. The law states: "No person in the United States shall, on the basis of sex, be excluded from participating in, be denied the benefits of, or be subjected to discrimination under any education program or activity receiving Federal Financial assistance" (fn 20 U.S.C. 1681 and 34 C.F.R. Part 106).

Initially, the emphasis of Title IX was the protection of equity in athletics. Later interpretations added attention to educational equity and access throughout single-sex and career/technical programs, and more recently specific protections for transgender (nonbinary) and pregnant or parenting students enrolled in publicly funded educational programs and services. Through a number of Supreme Court cases (fn *Franklin v. Gwinnet County*

Public Schools, 503 U.S. 60 (1992); *Gebser v. Lago Vista Indep. School*, 524 U.S. 274 [1998]; *Davis v. Monroe County Bd. of Educ.*, 526 U.S. 629 [1999]), the definition of gender-based or sex discrimination was expanded to include discrimination through incidents of sexual harassment and other kinds of sexual misconduct, the impact of which the court saw as also depriving a student of his or her educational opportunities.

As the Supreme Court found in *Davis v. Monroe Cty. Bd. of Educ*, when sexual misconduct is so severe, persistent, or pervasive as to deny or limit a student's ability to participate in or benefit from a school's programs or activities, a hostile environment exists and the school must respond. In furtherance of these decisions, the federal government has promulgated regulations and the United States Department of Education have issued Dear Colleague letters to provide guidance to schools on its responsibilities under Title IX.

Definitions of what constitutes sexual harassment vary and each school must consider the complicated nuances of problematic sexualized behavior and their impact on students' ability to feel safe while at school. Generally, Title IX considers sexual harassment as any form of sex discrimination when the behavior "can interfere with a student's academic performance and emotional and physical well-being" (OCR, 2001, p. ii), or in other words, the harassment creates a hostile environment.

One example of what is broadly prohibited by Title IX in a K–12 school is illustrated as follows:

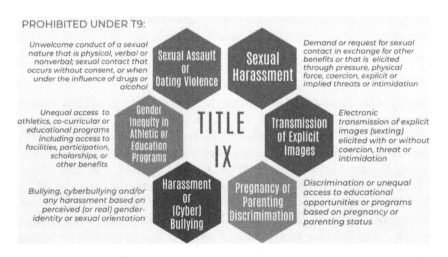

PROHIBITED UNDER T9:

Unwelcome conduct of a sexual nature that is physical, verbal or nonverbal; sexual contact that occurs without consent, or when under the influence of drugs or alcohol — **Sexual Assault or Dating Violence**

Sexual Harassment — Demand or request for sexual contact in exchange for other benefits or that is elicited through pressure, physical force, coercion, explicit or implied threats or intimidation

Unequal access to athletics, co-curricular or educational programs including access to facilities, participation, scholarships, or other benefits — **Gender Inequity in Athletic or Education Programs**

TITLE IX

Transmission of Explicit Images — Electronic transmission of explicit images (sexting) elicited with or without coercion, threat or intimidation

Bullying, cyberbullying and/or any harassment based on perceived (or real) gender-identity or sexual orientation — **Harassment or (Cyber) Bullying**

Pregnancy or Parenting Discrimimation — Discrimination or unequal access to educational opportunities or programs based on pregnancy or parenting status

In this example, the categories broadly described as sexual assault or dating violence, sexual harassment, transmission of explicit images, and harassment or cyberbullying are all variations of sexual harassment as delineated by Title IX.

THE FEDERAL FRAMEWORK

All educational agencies are required to designate at least one employee as a Title IX coordinator in charge of overseeing compliance within the agency; however, it is expected that the entire institution will share in this responsibility. At a minimum, the OCR requires a designated Title IX official responsible for "coordinating the implementation and administration of the recipient's procedures for resolving Title IX complaints, including educating the school community on how to file a complaint alleging a violation of Title IX, investigating complaints, working with law enforcement when necessary, and ensuring that complaints are resolved promptly and appropriately" (Lhamon, 2015, p. 2).

In addition to investigating all complaints of gender discrimination, schools must provide notice to students and employees of the name and contact information of the Title IX coordinator. This information must be visible, offered in a variety of modalities (online, in schools), and use clear language that children of all ages can understand. In some cases, this may require translation services, posted in languages other than English.

The Supreme Court decisions noted above caused the U.S. Department of Education to revise its guidance on Title IX. The January 2001 Dear Colleague letter sets out the framework which governs all Title IX investigations. Subsequent Dear Colleague letters from 2011, 2014, and most recently from 2017, have offered updates and amendments to the process.

In the 2014 Dear Colleague letter, the Obama administration specifically included protections against discrimination for transgender students. This guidance was rescinded by the Trump administration; however, some states, including Oregon, have determined to continue the protections afforded to transgender students and to uphold discrimination findings under Title IX.

The Oregon guidance directs Oregon educators to provide transgender students with access which allows them the freedom of choice in dress, preferred names and pronouns, use of lockers and restrooms, and so on. In addition, the guidance echoes the 2014 Dear Colleague letter's determination that gender-based discrimination is included within the meaning of discrimination on the basis of sex. https://www.oregon.gov/ode/students-and-family/equity/civilr ights/Documents/TransgenderStudentGuidance.pdf)

OFFICE OF CIVIL RIGHTS

The Office for Civil Rights of the U.S. Department of Education is responsible for Title IX enforcement. OCR is in charge of evaluating, investigating, and resolving complaints of school-based sex discrimination. As part of its purview, it may also conduct compliance reviews of educational institutions to investigate potential systemic violations.

Additionally, it has the authority to develop policy and compliance standards on the regulations it enforces. Under OCR compliance standards, when an educational agency has notice of an allegation of sexual harassment, it must immediately take appropriate steps to investigate the allegation. It is also required to provide interim measures to prevent further harm to the student, while an investigation is pending and to enact structural changes to remedy the effects and prevent its recurrence.

TITLE IX IN K–12

In 2001, the Office of Civil Rights published the Revised Sexual Harassment Guidance, which remains the most instructive for K–12 application. The underlying principle reflected in the publication is that "Preventing and remedying sexual harassment in schools is essential to ensuring a safe environment in which students can learn" (OCR, January 2001, p. ii). Behaviors that may create a hostile environment require the school immediately act to "end the harassment, prevent its recurrence" and, as appropriate, "remedy its effects" (OCR, p. iii).

For postsecondary education, the release of the 2014 Dear Colleague Letter, a "53-page document focused on procedural protections, confidentiality and responsible employee definitions, investigation and hearing protocol, interim measures, remedies and appeals, and training requirements" (O'Banion, 2018, p. 49) had a remarkable effect. While colleges and universities scrambled to create Title IX offices, appoint coordinators and implement new policies and procedures, K–12 schools were largely left out of the recommendations offered. While this may not have been intended by the Obama administration, K–12 schools did not see their unique environments reflected in guidance and emerging practice recommendations, thus, the 2001 revised guidance remains the most influential for K–12 administrators.

While SIRC is not an investigatory framework for comprehensive Title IX response, it does provide an option for safety planning specific to the child exhibiting problematic behaviors, which in turn can keep other children in the school community safe. SIRC offers a particularly useful tool for interim measures, and, when applied appropriately, can also play a role in remedying the effects on children in school. Interim measures, first defined by the 2001 federal guidance as "individualized services offered as appropriate to either or both the reporting and responding parties involved in an alleged incident of sexual misconduct, prior to an investigation or while an investigation is pending" (2001) was further clarified in 2017 with the release of OCR's Q&A on Sexual Misconduct.

The updated language about interim measures specifically delineated actions for interim safety such as "counseling, extensions of time or other course-related adjustments, modifications of work or class schedules, campus escort services, restrictions on contact between the parties, changes in work or housing locations, leaves of absence, increased security and monitoring of certain areas of campus, and other similar accommodations" (OCR, 2017, p. 2). Clearly, not all these examples are applicable to the K–12 landscape, however, many, such as schedule changes, no contact orders and flexibility of academic deadlines, are absolutely appropriate for K–12 schools. The following Venn diagram, used by Portland Public Schools, illustrates the necessary components of a comprehensive Title IX response framework.

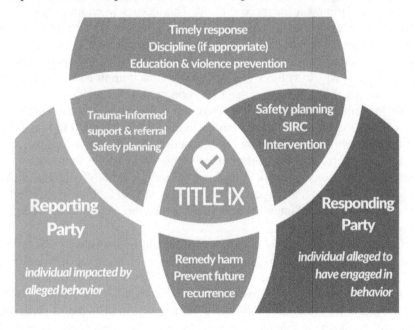

INVESTIGATIONS IN K–12 SCHOOLS

Not all incidents of problematic sexual behavior constitute sexual harassment under Title IX. OCR has cautioned K–12 schools not to overreact to what may be developmentally appropriate behavior, such as a kiss on the cheek by a young child (OCR, 2001) and encouraged "School personnel to consider the age and maturity of students in responding to allegations of sexual harassment" (OCR, 2001, p. iii). Broadly, the 2001 guidance outlined three types of sexual harassment complaint that would trigger a Title IX investigation: quid pro quo harassment; retaliatory harassment; and harassment that creates a hostile environment.

Quid pro quo harassment occurs when a school employee explicitly or implicitly conditions a student's participation in an educational program or makes an educational decision on that student's submission to sexual requests or advances, or any other verbal, nonverbal, or physical conduct of a sexual nature. Because of the nature of the staff/student relationship, this type of harassment is unlawful whether or not the student resists and suffers actual harm.

Retaliatory harassment occurs when an adverse action is taken against a person because of that person's participation, either as a complainant, a witness, or reporter, in a complaint of discrimination or sexual harassment.

The most prevalent type of harassment seen in the school setting is where a hostile environment has been created. This occurs when an employee or student engages in sexually harassing conduct, which can include unwelcome sexual advances, requests for sexual favors, and other verbal, nonverbal, or physical conduct of a sexual nature that is sufficiently severe, persistent, or pervasive and which is objectively offensive in that it limits a student's ability to participate in or benefit from an education program or activity.

In determining whether a hostile environment exists, the investigator must look at the totality of circumstances including, but not limited to, the effect of the behavior on the reporting party; whether the behavior was directed at one or more persons; whether the behavior unreasonably interfered with those persons' educational or work performances; and so on. For incidents of discriminatory or derogatory speech, investigators should look, as well, at what the statement was, its intention and whether there are any First Amendment protections in play.

Certain conduct, such as sexual assault, would be considered severe and would, in and of itself, constitute a hostile environment. In other instances, a pattern of pervasive or persistent behavior would need to be shown in order to satisfy the conditions of this finding. Pervasive conduct occurs in public places like the classroom or within the workplace. An example of pervasive conduct would be a school-wide acceptance (or at least complacency) of discriminatory treatment toward transgender students. Persistent conduct is repeated behavior or speech over a period of time that continues despite requests to stop. For example, the student who sexually harasses a fellow student on a daily basis despite clear signals from the student or others that this is unwelcome behavior.

Finally, proof that a hostile environment exists is satisfied by the objectively offensive standard as interpreted by a reasonable person. Factors include the age, vulnerability, and relationship of the parties; the number of persons involved; the frequency and severity of the behavior, the existence of violence or the threat of violence; resulting humiliation or ridicule toward the complainant. Hostile environment harassment requires further steps to assess whether or not the "conduct is sufficiently serious to deny or limit a student's ability to participate in, or benefit from, the school's program based on sex" (OCR, 2001, p. 5).

Analysis regarding the type, frequency, and duration of conduct, the degree to which the behavior was targeted at one or more students, the relationship between those involved, the number involved in the harassment, the age and sex of the harasser, the size, location and context in which the harassment occurred within the school, and whether the incident is sufficiently severe enough to create a hostile environment are also important considerations (OCR, 2001).

Determining whether any of the factors exists is central to the preliminary inquiry in which the investigator determines whether there is reasonable cause to open a formal investigation. This is also the time to reach out to the reporting party to better understand how the person is feeling and what he/she would like the process to be. It is best to approach this in a trauma-informed way and to provide this person with as much control in terms of their participation as possible. This is also the time to put into place interim safety measures to ensure that both parties are kept safe.

GRIEVANCE PROCEDURES

The creation and posting of grievance procedures poses a unique challenge within the K–12 system due to the vast continuum of parents, students, and community members' needs. Posting clear, developmentally and age-appropriate procedures in places that are easy to access is a challenge across K–12 schools. A poster about harassment and bullying that conveys the message well to high schoolers may not work for an elementary school. At a minimum, adopted grievance procedures must provide for prompt and equitable resolution of any complaint and include a districtwide policy against sex discrimination (OCR, 2001).

Kids must have a clear understanding of the kinds of incidents the school must respond to, what constitutes discrimination under Title IX, and perhaps most importantly, what happens once a complaint is made. Attention should be paid to the diversity of children and communities and the uniqueness of each school building when deciding how to post resolution procedures. They may need to vary even within the context of a single school district.

When schools fail to clearly delineate the complexities of the law, Title IX school policy and resulting procedures, additional harm or trauma may occur. A child who discloses to a trusted adult school staff member may believe they can do in a confidential manner, only later to find out that staff member is a mandatory reporter and must share the information with the Title IX coordinator. This can be experienced by the child (and their family) as retaliatory and when this is combined with feelings that the school ignores or acts against the wishes of someone who has been harmed, it has been closely linked with additional secondary harms suffered, and referred to in the literature as institutional betrayal (Gobin & Freyd, 2013; Goldsmith et al., 2012; Platt et al., 2009). Other manifestations of betrayal can include "indifferent policies which fail to protect, inaccessible reporting procedures, ineffective response by the university, or failure to redress harm" or "when institutions fail to act at all, dismiss a claim, or fail to protect a student from further harm or retaliation" (O'Banion, 2018, p. 70).

THE NEED FOR FORMAL INVESTIGATION

The school may decide to take appropriate interim measures while an investigation proceeds, including using SIRC for safety planning, adjusting class schedules or even suspending the student pending the disciplinary hearing or outcome. Regardless, if the school determines to proceed to a formal investigation, both the reporting and responding party must be notified both verbally and in writing. The notice should include the allegation, the policy or policies that have been implicated and the process by which the investigation will proceed with a projected timeline for completion. The notice should include how the investigation will work to maintain privacy. It may also include the interim actions identified by the SIRC coordinator for student-on-student incidents or by the Human Resources Department (for staff-on-student incidents). Practice varies by district as to whether parents and guardians are also noticed. Look to your district's policy for guidance.

Both parties are allowed to have an adviser to assist them during the course of the investigation. The adviser could include a parent or guardian, a school counselor, a union representative, or an attorney, to name a few. The adviser may accompany the party during the interview or later, at a hearing, but they may not, in most cases, speak on behalf of the party. There may be instances where the student's age or developmental disability requires the adviser to assist in answering questions on behalf of the student.

It is likely that parents or guardians will want to be completely involved in all aspects of the investigation. They have the right to inspect and review all educational records of the student under FERPA and this right extends to the investigation records that directly relate to their child. In the same way that the reporting and responding parties are advised of the investigation and discipline processes in play, the investigator should discuss these processes to them in order with help them understand and support their child.

While there may be instances where behavior is captured on video or through text messaging and other social media platforms, most investigations will rely on interviews. Best practice is to interview parties and witnesses as soon as possible while their recollections are fresh. It is also better to have a second person in the interview to help take notes. If that isn't possible, create a summary of the interview and then have the witness sign it confirming its accuracy. Witnesses may be identified by one or both parties and the investigator should assess the best order for interviewing them.

Once all of the interviews are completed and any other evidence gathered, the investigator must determine whether the evidence meets the evidentiary standard your district has determined is necessary in order to make a finding of Title IX violation. For many years, the standard of evidence was preponderance, in other words, it was "more likely than not" that the incident occurred. Under the Trump administration, schools and districts were given the option of retaining the preponderance standard or moving to the higher standard of clear and convincing evidence.

Most investigations should be completed quickly and delays such as school vacations or police investigations should be documented along with the evidence and interviews. If an extension is needed, both parties should be notified of the extension.

Once the investigation is completed, the investigator will prepare a report detailing the allegations, the names of the witnesses and other evidence gathered. The report should summarize the findings and the final determination made by the investigator. It should also include any remedial measures, such as no contact orders, that should be in place prior to the completion of the process. The report should be provided to both parties as well as to the person designated to adjudicate the matter.

The adjudicator should review the information provided by the investigator and listen to the testimony of the reporting and responding parties. While the law in this area is in flux, there is language in the guidance that each party has the right of cross-examination. One way to approach this is to use the adjudicator as the intermediary who asks questions on behalf of each party. Once the adjudicator has reviewed the report and heard from the parties, he or she will issue sanctions if the evidence meets the evidentiary threshold of preponderance or clear and convincing evidence. These sanctions are then included in the final report, a copy of which is provided to each party. Sanctions should be proportionate to the severity of the behavior. In cases of adult on student misconduct, schools should also be cognizant of employee protections found in state law.

Both parties have a right to appeal the final order and so each district should have an appeal process in addition to the investigatory process outlined in this chapter. Following a determination that sexual harassment occurred, there are two requirements to fully address the harassment. First, the school must determine a "reasonable, timely, age-appropriate, and effective corrective action, including steps tailored to the specific situation" (OCR, 2001, p. 16). Lastly, steps must be taken to prevent future recurrence. This protects both parties from retaliation and any witnesses involved in the fact-finding portion of the investigation. There may also be a need to continue to monitor the behavior of the harasser, refer them to educational or counseling options, and/or other scheduled times for follow-up or check-in to ensure the behavior has stopped.

Chapter 10

Special Considerations and Unusual Situations

Given the nature of this work, you will always be amazed at the unusual situations you encounter. This chapter was included for the purpose of helping you to avoid common pitfalls, and so that you can further develop your own thinking with regard to how to address these problems. Being good at addressing problematic sexual behavior is not about book smarts. Rather, it's about keeping a cool head and using common sense.

MASTURBATION

Masturbation is a topic most people would rather not discuss. It's one of those behaviors that everyone engages in, but most people deny doing. It is considered sinful by some and shameful by many. Since you are part of the human race, I've no doubt that you were likely raised with some hang-ups about this behavior, and it's likely those hang-ups have impacted your views on this topic. You should be aware that this topic is also really hard for your students and their parents.

Whatever your personal or religious views on the topic, it's important that you understand that masturbation is considered a normal part of healthy human development by physicians, psychologists, and the scientific community. That being said, your goal should not be to stamp it out at any cost through shaming kids, but rather to make sure that it happens in an environment where it is considered acceptable (i.e., in the privacy of their home bathroom or bedroom) rather than in your school. In order for this plan to work, you'll need to get the students' parents on board. If you can't be the one to do it because of your beliefs about masturbation, please help your students and their families by connecting them to a professional in your community who does not have negative, unrealistic, or outmoded views about masturbation.

I've found that normalizing the behavior is a great way to diffuse the anxiety parents have around this topic: "You see, Mr. Jones, masturbation and curiosity about one's body is a normal part of human development. I'm not suggesting that your son stop doing this; rather, I want to make sure that he knows where he can and can't engage in this behavior. Is there somewhere in the house that you could let him know would be an okay place for him to do this in private?"

PREPUBESCENT FEMALES AND MASTURBATION

This is a surprisingly common behavioral phenomenon that can take many forms. In some cases, girls will rub their genitals against furniture, the floor, a pillow, or some other object. Some will use their hand to stimulate themselves, while others possess the unique gift of being able to stimulate themselves hands-free (usually by rubbing their thighs together). Sometimes the behavior is so pronounced that everyone in the class notices it, and sometimes it's so subtle that even a well-trained teacher can have trouble detecting it.

Many people, when first encountering this behavior, make the hasty assumption that the girl engaging in this behavior has been sexually victimized. While sexual victimization is an important possibility to consider, there are other possibilities to cross off your list first.

You should start by first looking for a medical explanation. It's possible that all the rubbing you are seeing is the result of an itch, due to an infection, or some other medical problem. So, if you see this behavior at school, start by encouraging the parents to take their child for a medical evaluation.

It should also be noted that many girls develop masturbatory behavior completely on their own, without any inappropriate exposure to adult sexual behavior. It's not uncommon to see this behavior in kindergarteners, and I've run across cases where parents described that their daughter developed the ability to masturbate before she could walk.

Girls who develop this ability on their own typically do not view the behavior as sexual in nature, and they do not evidence any interest in or knowledge about adult sexual behavior. To them, this is simply a neat trick that feels great and helps to relieve the boredom. It has absolutely nothing to do with sex as far as they are concerned. Your goal, when you see it show up in your school, is to help them and their parents understand that the behavior is fine provided it's done in privacy at their own home and not in public or while at school.

Please note that you may find the behavior particularly difficult to extinguish and it may be useful to employ some creative classroom strategies designed to interrupt the behavior (like distraction). Do not waste your time attempting to develop a reward-based strategy (i.e., sticker chart) around extinguishing the behavior. Star charts, M&M's, and extra time at recess just don't hold a candle to orgasm. There is no greater reward for human beings. It's how we're hardwired. There wouldn't be seven billion people on the planet if this weren't the case.

FREQUENT VAGINAL INFECTIONS

As just mentioned, sometimes what appears to be masturbation is just physical discomfort brought on by a vaginal infection or other medical problem. But please also be on the lookout for girls who continually have problems with this part of their anatomy. Sometimes frequent vaginal infections can be the result of irritating soaps or bubble bath. Unfortunately, however, recurrent problems in this area can sometimes be the result of sexual abuse. Whatever the cause, it's important that it not be ignored, and that you make sure the child is being evaluated by a physician. Remember, refusing to provide adequate medical care for a child can be the basis for filing a report with your local Child Protective Services.

VAMPIRES, WEREWOLVES, WITCHES, AND MORE

Remember when vampires were creepy? Unfortunately, with the advent of books like *Twilight* and card games like Magic: The Gathering, these once frightening folk have become the icons for our lost and disaffected youth. Don't be surprised if you unearth (pun fully intended) your own little coven or tribe or whatever the heck they call themselves at your school.

Within the context of problematic sexual behavior, pretending to be a vampire or having involvement in the occult is an unusual but effective strategy for middle school and high school students to organize group sexual behavior. Typically, the orgiastic engagements are orchestrated by one or two sophisticated kids who have surrounded themselves with an impressionable and less sophisticated flock.

Considering that you may have multiple individuals involved in such an incident, supervision/intervention planning can be particularly challenging. Generally speaking, the best strategy when addressing this type of group behavior is divide and conquer. Make sure that your supervision plans include no contact orders between the offending parties while at school and encourage parents to prohibit their children from having contact with their fellow bloodsuckers while in the community.

PEDOPHILES

Pedophilia is commonly defined as sexual interest in children (usually children under the age of thirteen). But in truth it is much more than that. Pedophilia includes the romantic interest in children as well. It may not seem like an important distinction, but it is, because most child molesters are not pedophiles. Yeah—read that last sentence again. It's not a typo.

Although there is some debate, scientific research suggests that people who molest children can generally be broken up into two groups: pedophiles (those who are romantically and sexually interested in kids) and non-pedophilic child molesters (individuals who evidence sexual and romantic interest in adults but offend kids for other reasons).

As soon as you read the word *pedophile*, you probably thought about some creepy old man hiding out in the bushes of some seedy park, waiting to prey on children. But research suggests that a good percentage of adjudicated pedophiles got their start when they were young, which means that there are very likely some future pedophiles running around your school right now. Don't panic.

Although you will encounter a host of unusual sexual behaviors in your school district, a very small percentage of these behaviors will be committed by pedophiles, because they are relatively rare. While there are no reliable base rates or estimations about the prevalence of pedophilia in the general population, in serving a district with over 40,000 students in an urban setting, one might routinely encounter about 150 to 200 cases of problematic sexual behavior a year. Of those cases, maybe eight to nine would qualify as pedophilic.

Please remember it's not your job to identify or diagnose pedophiles. Rather, it's your job to seek consultation on any case that you consider to be too complex. If you make sure to seek consultation when you see concerning grooming behavior or targeted sexual behavior toward children that does not remit with intervention, you can sleep well at night knowing that you are doing everything in your power to keep your school and your community safe.

SEXUALLY REACTIVE BEHAVIOR

By and large, the majority of the kids who evidence problematic sexual behavior in school are best described as children with sexually reactive behavior.

These are kids who experienced some troubling premature exposure to adult sexual behavior that left them confused, anxious, and sexually aroused. Some of these kids were sexually molested, some of these kids found their older brother's pornography stash, some of these kids live in sexualized environments with poor boundaries around sexual behavior, and the list goes on.

Most of these kids are pretty anxious about their sexual behavior and what they need most is help making sense out of what they experienced. It's not your job to help them with this, but it is your job to connect them to a helpful community resource so that their problematic sexual behavior can be addressed before it becomes more harmful. You can do this with the help of your school counselor or access assistance from your Level 2 team.

PSYCHOPATHS

Psychopaths are individuals who have no reservation about violating social norms for their own gratification. They have little regard for the welfare of others and they can present as cunning, manipulative, and charismatic. These individuals are frequently described as impulsive thrill seekers with no moral compass. This is another group where there are fortunately very few in your schools.

Thought of within the context of problematic sexual behavior, these individuals have little concern about using force and coercion with their victims, and they feel no genuine remorse for their behavior or empathy for the individuals they harm. Some of these individuals will present with a host of other concerning behaviors that include lying, theft, and assault. They evidence little regard for authority figures and appear to delight in rule breaking.

Oftentimes, these types of individuals have a history of harming animals, and other individuals over whom they have power. They are incredibly dangerous, and when you see a student evidencing these types of behaviors you should set up a very restrictive supervision plan and seek consultation with your Level 2 team immediately.

If you are responsible for crafting the intervention plan for a student who fits the description used above, it is important to remember a few things. First, you should know that these types of individuals often are more cued in to the emotional response they receive from others than they are the consequences of their actions. In other words, these types of kids aren't nearly as concerned with the consequences of their actions (punishment/reward) as they are about how you emotionally respond to them.

Consequently, it will be important to help teachers and instructional assistants understand that they will have more success when they deliver unemotional positive and negative consequences to this type of child. No huge celebrations of success, and no drawn-out lectures when bad behavior occurs. Just simple consequences delivered without fanfare. You do A behavior you get B consequence. The goal in working with these individuals is to reward them for demonstrating compliance with supervision and skills training should be attempted with caution, as it can often make them more dangerous to others.

MENTAL ILLNESS

In some cases, problematic sexual behavior in children may co-occur with, or be an artifact of, mental illness. Children who are losing touch with reality, experiencing a psychotic break, reexperiencing trauma, or are overly ruminative may exhibit problematic sexual behavior that is a manifestation of their psychological disturbance. Generally, this type of problematic sexual behavior is bizarre and confusing in its presentation, and the child will generally evidence a host of other unusual, disorganized, and disturbing behaviors that may serve to alert you to their mental state.

Helping these children connect to mental health services will be an important part of the intervention strategy employed to help them. Again, you can do this via your school counselor or via your Level 2 team depending upon the resources available to you.

AUTISM SPECTRUM

Autistic children are often the source of much fearful (and misguided) speculation in school districts. All too frequently teachers or administrators will call in a panic, worried about the next "Kip Kinkel" or "Jeffrey Dahmer," who on further investigation turns out to be a relatively typical student with Autism Spectrum Disorder (ASD). Oftentimes, the poor social reciprocity aspect that is a hallmark of the autism spectrum is misinterpreted as antisocial rather than asocial. This is not to suggest that kids on the autism spectrum lack the capacity to harm others; rather, that being on the autism spectrum does not increase the likelihood that a child will engage in harmful behavior toward others.

With regard to their sexual development, very little is known about kids on the autism spectrum. There are a handful of scientific papers on this topic, and clearly a need for additional research. That being said, you will likely find that kids on the autism spectrum do occasionally exhibit unusual sexual behaviors at school that may lead to a need for additional supervision. On the one hand, problematic sexual behavior in children with ASD can be challenging to change because these children tend to be somewhat more ruminative in their thinking. However, their commitment to rule-following can often make them somewhat more easy to supervise, as long as their supervision plan is very concrete with regard to expectations, and it will help to have an ASD specialist in the room when developing the supervision plan.

Generally speaking, problematic sexual behavior among autistic kids tends to be the by-product of some sort of sexual fixation. In part, this is likely due to the fact that, in comparison to neurotypicals (or children without autism), kids on the autism spectrum are more ruminative and obsessional about a variety of topics. It just makes sense that their sexual development would also reflect this same tendency toward fixation.

Sometimes the sexual fixation is on a behavior, sometimes it falls on an object, and sometimes it falls on a specific person. In some cases, this fixation can cause the student to behave in ways that are suggestive of stalking behavior, and it's not uncommon that this is how the behavior first comes to the attention of others.

The other group of common problematic sexual behaviors exhibited by kids on the autism spectrum tends to be related to poor understanding of socially normative behavior. These kids may make their peers and teachers uncomfortable because they don't seem to understand how to regulate or contain their sexual behavior in socially appropriate ways. Whatever the domain, you will likely benefit from consultation with an autism specialist in your district in order to develop an effective intervention.

If you are the autism specialist in your district, you may find that many of the same strategies you put into place when attempting to modify or extinguish other concerning behaviors with autism spectrum kids also works with regard to modifying their sexual behavior. With a little creativity, social stories, token economies, and PECS (Picture Exchange Communication System) boards can be used toward that end.

Please be aware, however, that extinguishing problematic sexual behavior may prove more challenging than extinguishing hand-flapping or improving eye contact. Sexual behavior carries its own reward (sexual pleasure), and one that is far more powerful than a sticker chart or a Pokémon card. Consequently, you will likely need to employ multiple interventions simultaneously at home and at school if you hope to change the behavior.

You may also find it helpful to consult with a mental health professional with a background in sexual behavior or sexual misconduct when developing intervention strategies. There is some evidence in the literature that sexual behaviors can be shaped via complex behavior modification strategies, but it is recommended that these only be attempted by trained professionals.

COGNITIVE IMPAIRMENT

Students with serious cognitive impairment are often overlooked with regard to the problematic sexual behavior they exhibit because people regard the behavior as "harmless"; they feel they don't know what to do about the behavior, and/or they believe that the student "can't help it." Ignoring this behavior does not make it go away, however, and allowing it to continue only creates a feeling of discomfort and unsafety in the classroom.

There was a case many years ago in which the family of a child with serious cognitive impairment had started accommodating their child's masturbatory behavior anywhere in the house (the behavior had started bleeding into the school). Although the parents were very loving and concerned about their child's welfare, they had not thought through the potential problems this would create for their child over the course of her life.

When it was brought to their attention that this behavior would not be tolerated in a group home, they expressed their confidence that their child would be living at home with them during her adult life. They seemed surprised when I pointed out that their child was in great health and would likely outlive them by a span of thirty years or more, at which point she would be expected to change a behavior she had been engaging in for a very long time. Clearly, they meant well. They just hadn't factored their own mortality into their daughter's long-term plan. Ultimately, they got on board and accepted the fact that this behavior was going to have to be changed.

The Level 1 and Level 2 system can be used just as successfully with this population as with your cognitively intact students. The Level 1 protocol can be used to open a discussion about the problematic sexual behavior with the important individuals who best know the student, and any complicated cases that require further consultation can be forwarded to your Level 2 team.

In developing intervention and supervision strategies for this population, it's important to note that it will require focused and sustained intervention to bring about behavior change. As mentioned previously, behavioral strategies that rely on rewards and punishments may not be impactful given the powerful intrinsic reward of sexual pleasure. That being said, it may be more reasonable to attempt to relocate the problematic sexual behavior to a more appropriate place and time (provided that the behavior is not assaultive) rather than try to extinguish it altogether.

FIRE SETTING

There was a time when all fire-setting behavior was believed to be a form of sexual perversion. Nowadays, that notion has largely been debunked by researchers and clinicians. Fire-setting behavior is now thought to stem from multiple sources, including (but not limited to) curiosity, conduct issues, psychopathy, and mental illness.

Although fire-setting is no longer believed to be a form of sexual perversion, there are rare but documented cases of pyrophilia (sexual fascination with fire) and instances in which fire-setting has played a role in problematic sexual behavior.

If you encounter a blend of problematic sexual behavior and fire setting, it is important that in addition to following your protocol for addressing problematic sexual behavior you also seek to address the fire-setting behavior. So, as you are sending this case along to your Level 2 team, you should also be contacting your local fire department to seek their advice regarding how best to proceed.

Also, please keep in mind that if you ever discover evidence of a fire, after extinguishing the fire, do not clean up the evidence of the fire. Oftentimes, fire investigators can learn a great deal about how a fire occurred and who set the fire provided that the evidence is not disturbed.

AGGRESSIVE SEXUAL BEHAVIOR

Aggressive sexual behavior refers to any type of romantic or sexualized behavior that appears hostile, aggressive, or coercive. At its most extreme, aggressive sexual behavior can manifest as rape, which I think everyone can agree is a very bad thing. In less extreme forms, however, aggressive sexual behavior can be much harder to pin down.

Walk the halls of any high school during passing period and you will notice a number of happy couples innocently kissing or snuggling in the hallways. Most of these kids seem pretty blissful. But keep looking and it won't take you long to spot the not-so-happy couple.

He's got her trapped against her locker, speaking quiet, and controlled. She looks terrified. Teachers and staff tend to walk right on by these couples and not say a thing. It's understandable. Who wants to get into the middle of that?

While it would be ridiculous to suggest that the boy or girl engaging in this type of coercive behavior is a rapist, it does seem obvious that this type of behavior is a form of sexualized aggression. As such, it should always be confronted when identified, and considered legitimate grounds for a Level 1 protocol. Also, it should be noted that sexualized aggression occurs among LGBTQIA+ kids as well, and that sometimes it's a female aggressing against a male, so it's important to be attuned to this type of behavior regardless of gender.

VIOLENT THREAT

As noted in the section above, sometimes problematic sexual behavior has a violent element to it as well. Students who threaten or engage in rape, or are otherwise sexually assaultive, are not only engaging in problematic sexual behavior but also engaging in violent behavior. Consequently, interventions and supervision strategies for these individuals need to consider not only the sexual elements but also the potentially violent elements of their behavior.

If your district is fortunate enough to have a team that specializes in evaluating violent threat, it is important to include that team in your discussions regarding how best to mitigate risk and craft an intelligent intervention. Obviously, this can most easily be accomplished by including your Level 2 team. If your district does not have a threat assessment team or a Level 2 team, it would be wise to include law enforcement officials or violent threat assessment professionals in your intervention discussion.

LESBIAN/GAY/BISEXUAL/TRANSGENDERED/ QUEER/INTERSEX/ASEXUAL/ALLIES+ (LGBTQIA+)

Not unlike masturbation, homosexuality is a topic about which many people have opinions. Regardless of your own personal beliefs about it, there is abundant research literature indicating that homosexuality is a normal variation in sexual expression seen among many different species of animals, homo sapiens included. Although there was once a time where homosexuality was viewed as sexually deviant and psychologically unhealthy, scientific research has since disproved these outmoded notions.

In spite of what scientists now recognize about homosexuality, there remains a sizeable contingent of individuals who continue to feel strongly that it is morally wrong. On occasion, some of these individuals have taken steps to deny freedoms to LGBTQIA+ kids (not allowing them to attend school dances, refusing them the right to form school clubs, etc.).

Although there was once a time where this type of discrimination went unnoticed, this is no longer the case. If you are among the group of individuals who feels strongly that homosexuality is wrong, it is important that you understand that discriminating against LGBTQIA+ youth on the basis of sexual orientation or gender identity is no longer tolerated and will likely be met with civil lawsuits. It's also just plain mean. If you engage in this type of discriminatory behavior, you will make headlines, and not in a good way.

When you encounter a student in your school who is in the process of coming out as LGBTQIA+, or is being outed by someone at school, it is in everyone's best interest if you handle the situation as compassionately as possible. Encourage staff and parents to be supportive of the student, and encourage families and friends to access support via counseling, organizations like Parents, Families and Friends of Lesbians and Gays (www.pflag. org), and websites like It Gets Better Project (www.itgetsbetter.org).

It is to everyone's benefit to treat LGBTQIA+ kids the same way you treat your other students. Besides being the moral thing to do, it will also keep your district from getting its pants sued off. Afford these students the same rights and privileges enjoyed by your heterosexual students, but also be mindful to hold them to the same expectations. It's just as wrong to extend extra privileges as it is to deny them. If you are made aware of problematic sexual behavior, whether it be homosexual or heterosexual, you need to consider it and respond to it with the same even hand. All that being said, SIRC is not a tool for outing and/or harassing LGBTQIA+ kids.

While we are on the topic, a quick note about language. The term *homosexual* is considered unsavory by many individuals because it is thought to be overly clinical sounding and because it doesn't accurately represent the variation of sexual expression that needs to be considered and protected. Generally speaking, the terms *lesbian, gay, bisexual, transgendered, queer, intersex*, and *asexual* are thought to be more respectful and politically correct. The term *queer* is also commonly used by some individuals to describe themselves; however, this is a term you may want to shy away from as it also has negative and humiliating connotations for some.

One other very important thing. You will encounter cases in SIRC where problematic sexual behavior occurs between children of the same sex, and/or with children who identify as LGBTQIA+. When this happens, it is vital to remember that the situation you encountered tells us nothing about the gender identity or sexual orientation of the children involved in the behavior. We must be vigilant about communicating this when we talk to the parents of the children involved in the behavior. As you likely know, many people carry serious prejudice against LGBTQIA+ kids and adults, and it's not helpful to anyone to consider the situation you encountered as an opportunity to "out" a child to his/her parents or community. You will need to tread very lightly with families when helping them work through these situations and take into account all the potential risk factors to the school, community, and children in the SIRC process when addressing these concerns. Remember, it is your duty to protect the reputation of the children you identify through SIRC.

FETISH/PARTIALISM

Fetish is a word used to describe sexual desire that is focused more on an object than on an individual. *Partialism* is a word used to describe sexual desire that is focused on a body part (like feet or hands). People with fetish-istic interest have been found to sexualize any number of things, including but not limited to shoes, underwear, leather, rubber, latex, riding crops, and gloves.

There is considerable debate in the literature regarding how healthy or unhealthy this behavior is. While there is increasing acceptance of fetishistic interest in mainstream society, there remains some clinical evidence that in a small subset of cases, fetishistic interest can be very unhealthy and a sign of disturbing psychopathology.

You might think of it the same way you think about First Person Shooter video games. The overwhelming majority of people who play these games do not commit violent crimes, but for a very small subset of individuals, gaming of this nature appears to accompany remarkable pathology.

I mention fetish here because it would be wise to be on the lookout for it. In some cases, individuals will assault others to get their object of interest. There was a fellow who had a thing for sweaty sandals at the college where I did my graduate work. He'd walk around college campuses searching for girls in Birkenstock sandals, whom he would then tackle so he could run off with their shoes.

Another guy used to break into people's homes so he could steal their underwear. It's a strange world we live in. It's important you know how strange, so that when you encounter these types of problematic sexual behav-iors you can approach them from the correct perspective, see them for the problematic sexual behavior that they are, and not just pass the behavior off as weird.

SEXTING

This discussion would be incomplete without a section on sexting. Sexting refers to a relatively recent cultural phenomenon in which mostly high school and college age students send each other graphic sexual pictures of themselves. While there is considerable evidence that this behavior is more a passing fad than a crisis of epic proportions, there are some things to consider when addressing it.

Although in most cases, this behavior is likely more akin to the mooning or streaking that occurred on high school and college campuses when we were kids, when a person under the age of eighteen takes a picture of their naked body and sends it to someone else, this can create a number of problems. Although most states have enacted laws to avoid prosecuting this type of behavior as child pornography, these images do sometimes end up online and are used as just that. Also, the sharing of these images creates disruption at school and is sometimes used to bully or coerce others. Sometimes, sexting is a symptom of a more serious problematic sexual behavior that warrants clinical attention. Whatever the case, SIRC is a great tool for examining the seriousness of this problem.

While not generally the case, one must also consider that sexting is sometimes used as a mechanism to coerce, groom, or sexually intimidate others. For example, unsavory individuals will often first convince a child to share a picture of themselves in their underwear and then threaten to send the photo out to their parents and friends, if more explicit photos or sexual behavior is not provided. Consequently, when you encounter this behavior in your school, please give thought to the way in which this behavior is being implemented. Does it appear to be a prank, misguided romantic behavior between two mutually interested kids, or is it being used as a mechanism for harm? Again, if you can't figure it out, send it along to your Level 2 team so that they can examine it more closely.

PORNOGRAPHY

Before we get to what to look for and how to deal with it, it's important to have a brief discussion about how pornography has changed since the intervention of the Internet. It used to be that pornography was primarily distributed via stores set up specifically for that purpose. If you wanted to access porn, you had to go to that sleazy store, risk the possibility of your car being identified out front of the store, risk the chance of being seen by someone you know inside, and then face the cashier as you made your purchase.

One can't help but think those shame-inducing factors prevented a number of people who would have liked to view pornography not only from purchasing it, but also from making purchases that might be viewed by others as particularly odd or deviant. This is not the world we currently live in.

Nowadays, anyone can go online and anonymously view an astonishingly wide variety of pornography. It doesn't matter how unusual your sexual proclivity, you can find it online, along with a chat group or discussion forum focused around that niche, and no one has to know about it.

Into clowns? Get off on balloon animals? How about sexy pie fights? It's all there for your viewing pleasure. While it's beyond the scope of this book to debate the merits of this all-access sexual pass with regard to the adult use of pornography, there is no question that the easy accessibility of pornography is uniformly a bad thing for children, as it often leads to problematic sexual behavior.

With regard to schools, one must make every effort to limit access to pornography through the Internet. Do not make the mistake of trusting your IT department to be solely responsible for this task. There are a myriad of ways around even the most sophisticated security systems, and so you must also encourage staff and parents to be vigilant about monitoring Internet usage, and you should be thoughtful with regard to the placement of your computer monitors such that they aid supervision.

Additionally, be on the lookout for kids in possession of pornography and thoughtful to the fact that pornography is often used in grooming children for sexual behavior. It works like this: Billy brings pornography to school to show Steve, in the hopes that getting Steve aroused will encourage Steve to participate in sexual behavior. It can be pretty insidious.

So, when you encounter a student who is bringing porn to school or viewing it at school on technology, it's perfectly reasonable to include regular searches and limit unsupervised access to technology (including cell phones) as part of a supervision/intervention plan. Further, if you have evidence suggesting that a student is using pornography to groom others, it would be wise to pass this referral along to your Level 2 team as grooming behavior is strongly suggestive of well-entrenched and problematic sexual behavior.

PARAPHILIC BEHAVIOR

Paraphilia literally means "other love." It is a term that refers broadly to unusual sexual behavior and includes, but is not limited to, pedophilia, sexual fetish, exhibitionism, voyeurism, zoophilia (bestiality), necrophilia (sex with dead people), sadism, masochism, and frotteurism (rubbing one's sexual parts against an object or person). While the majority of these behaviors are thought to be relatively rare, and some have gained a degree of cultural acceptance (sadism and masochism, for example), many paraphilias (necrophilia, pedophilia, zoophilia, to name a few) are associated with significant behavioral, psychological, and sexual pathology. Consequently, when you unearth evidence of these types of unusual sexual interests in your students, further examination is generally warranted.

A WORD FROM THE DISTRICT ATTORNEYS

I wasn't able to talk DDA's Brendan Murphy, JD, and David Wilson, JD, into writing a chapter for this book, however, they did provide some useful thoughts about how SIRC interfaces with the DA's office. Both agreed that although most juvenile justice systems are well equipped to address problematic sexual behavior in children thirteen years of age and older, "juveniles under the age of 12 are typically not of an appropriate level of development to be served by the juvenile justice system," and that "the Juvenile Dependency System is often better suited to address issues related to problematic sexual behavior than the Delinquency System because of the family dynamic usually seen in these cases." Further, although "there are cases where a juvenile who is 12 years old or younger is of an adequate developmental level so that the juvenile justice system can address his or her needs; the DDA & Juvenile department typically consult to determine whether a juvenile is sophisticated enough for juvenile justice system intervention to be appropriate."

Think back to the end of chapter 2 where we examined the pie charts (remember it showed that there are lots of Level 1 cases in elementary schools but that most of these cases don't go on to require Level 2 consultation). SIRC is well suited to address these challenging, under the age of twelve, cases that the juvenile department is unable to handle. This means that, through SIRC, you can get attention, services, supervision, and intervention to kids that are demonstrating problematic sexual behavior, but who would otherwise be ignored. Although this is still a reactive, rather than proactive, approach, having a school-based system in place allows us to respond to lower-level cases when the problematic behavior is just surfacing and when it is easier to change.

The DA's mentioned that SIRC has been a useful tool for helping reluctant families get on board with providing supervision and intervention to their children. SIRC does an excellent job of putting parents on notice, and specifically articulating the parental role in keeping the community safe from problematic sexual behavior their child may be exhibiting. At the end of a good Level 1 (or Level 2 if it gets that far), parents will know exactly what the school is recommending with regard to their child's supervision needs in the community and failure to follow through with these recommendations can be the basis for involving Child Protection Services. From this perspective, SIRC is a helpful tool to the DA's office as well.

Chapter 11

Extending the Model

Rural Settings, College Campuses, and Adults

The multileveled threat assessment response was developed for implementation in an urban public school setting, to be used with children who are exhibiting problematic sexual behavior. That said, since the publication of the first edition of this book, SIRC has been adapted for rural settings, and it could easily be adapted for college campuses, and even to address problematic sexual behavior in adults. The following are some things to consider in adapting this model to other contexts.

RURAL SETTINGS

Rural settings generally suffer from a lack of resources that urban settings do not. While there are fewer children to consider or be concerned about, there are also fewer law enforcement officers, fewer DHS workers, and fewer treatment providers. In spite of these limitations, rural settings also have some pronounced strengths. Due to the poverty of resources, rural schools are often well partnered with community members and local agencies as a result of need.

Few rural environments have the resources, much less the need, for a weekly threat assessment meeting geared toward problematic sexual behavior. As such, it may work better to have Level 2 meetings once a month or every three weeks, depending upon the need, or to only convene a Level 2 when there is need to do so. It may also help to combine your Level 2 meeting into an already existing meeting that involves the same community partners. For example, if you already have a functioning threat assessment team designed to address concerning violent threats, you may want to weave this model into that preexisting meeting. This is the approach they take in the district where my wife oversees threat response (they have around 7,000 kids in the district), and it seems to work very well.

Another effective strategy is to develop a Level 2 team by combining resources with neighboring rural districts. You may not have the need or the ability to host a regular Level 2 meeting, but by joining forces with other small neighboring districts you may find that this model is more manageable when the cost and responsibility is shared. Again, in my wife's district, nearby smaller districts will piggyback onto their Level 2 team as needed.

Finally, if your district is geographically close to a much larger district with greater resources, it may be that you can reach an arrangement with the larger district that would allow you to utilize the expertise of their Level 2 team on an as-needed basis. By partnering in such a fashion, your district would in essence receive the support, expertise, and much-needed liability sharing at a cost that may be more manageable than attempting to establish a Level 2 meeting independently.

COLLEGES AND UNIVERSITIES

As president of Noname University, Rudy has had to work through some pretty challenging situations. Recently though, he's met a situation that is causing him to lose a great deal of sleep. Andy is a freshman at NU with outstanding academic performance. Unfortunately, he's been repeatedly accused of sexual assault in the four months since his enrollment.

It appears that Andy hangs out at parties, both on and off campus, looking for young women who appear inebriated to sexually assault. Several students have come forward to voice their concerns about Andy, but thus far no victims have reported being sexually assaulted. Rudy knows that even if a victim were to report Andy for sexual assault, it's unlikely that Andy would face charges because situations where alcohol is involved make these cases very tricky. Rudy is very concerned about the safety of the students on his campus and uncertain how best to proceed.

It shouldn't surprise anyone that some children with problematic sexual behavior grow up and go off to college. These young men and women are much more difficult to detect and manage in a collegiate setting where students are afforded tremendous autonomy and very little supervision. When alcohol use and poor supervision are added to the mix, it's not surprising that close to one in four women will be the victim of a sexual assault prior to graduation.

A small fraction of the sexual assaults that occur on college campuses actually end up in criminal charges of any sort. Many are unreported and of those that are reported, many are "handled" by the university administrators rather than involving law enforcement. Because this is a domain in which few have expertise, school administrators vary in their capacity to successfully address problematic sexual behavior in their student body. As a result, they make decisions based on their best judgment that potentially leave their university open to liability and their student body exposed to threat.

Imagine if Rudy had a Level 1 protocol and Level 1 team to help him address his concerns. With a Level 1 team, Rudy would have a systematized methodology for determining how serious the problem was, as well as a means for putting some limitations on Andy's behavior. If NU had a Level 2 team, or shared a Level 2 team with the local school district, Rudy would also have a means for accessing consultation on difficult cases and a mechanism for spreading liability. Clearly, Rudy could sleep much better at night knowing that he was doing everything possible to protect the students at his school from further assault, while helping Andy to get some professional help regarding his sexual behavior.

In order to make the transition to the collegiate domain, the Level 1 protocol would require a few adaptations. For example, one would need to examine the Level 1 questions in order to make sure that they retain their relevance. It is unlikely that "grooming behaviors" are going to be very relevant on a college campus; neither will questions about targeting cognitively or developmentally delayed peers.

You will probably, however, want to add some questions about targeting peers who are otherwise incapacitated as a result of substance use. Be thoughtful to the situations you encounter on your campus, develop the Level 1 protocol using a multidisciplinary approach with some feedback from agencies in your area, and you can feel confident in the decisions that come from using the tool. It seems like a simple application, but having provided consultations to universities, there is a notable fascination among college administrators to "admire the problem" but seemingly very little interest in enacting any real-world changes.

When developing a Level 2 team at the collegiate level, universities can connect to community agencies in the same fashion I recommended to school districts, or you can partner with a local school district and share the Level 2 team, or. . .

ADULTS

Or a university could partner with a community-based Level 2 team that is designed to address problematic sexual behavior in adults. Here's how that might work.

Many cities around the nation have developed multidisciplinary/ multiagency threat assessment teams that are designed to identify adults who intend to harm others and provide intervention strategies to decrease harm. These teams track concerns as intimate as interpersonal violence (think: preventing domestic violence and threats made to loved ones) as well as threats on a much larger scale (think: preventing the next Oklahoma City bombing).

Typically, an adult threat assessment team is made up of individuals from local law enforcement, district attorneys' offices, community mental health, adult parole/probation, domestic violence organizations, state police, universities and community colleges, as well as other agencies that may have access to useful information pertaining to the assessment of violent threat. Extending this model to include the threat of sexual misconduct would involve adding relevant parole and probation professionals and someone with expertise in addressing problematic sexual behavior in adults.

An adult sexual threat assessment team could function as a part of a regular adult threat assessment team or it could function separately. Whatever the case, the scope and purpose of an adult sexual threat assessment team would be very similar to a regular adult threat assessment team except that the focus would be on problematic sexual threats and problematic sexual behavior of adults in the community.

Specifically, the adult sexual threat assessment team would meet on a regular basis to discuss concerning and threatening sexual behavior of adults in the community at large and develop intervention strategies to improve public safety. Got a registered sex offender that just moved into the area? How about a creepy neighborhood fellow who's been approaching kids in the park for help finding his lost puppy? College freshman who is sexually victimizing drunk girls at the local sorority house? Student at the community college who recently threatened to rape his teacher? The adult sexual threat assessment team could act as a consultation body, providing guidance and interventions for a host of concerning adult sexual behaviors and thereby improving public safety.

Appendix A

Level 1 Protocol

Please note, the Level 1 protocol was developed via a series of multiagency team meetings that took place at Salem-Keizer School District. The resulting document is a reflection of the thinking of that team. That being said, it is important to recognize that it is not an empirically validated risk prediction or assessment tool. Rather, it is a tool designed to capture important elements when considering risk and supervision issues for kids with concerning sexual behavior toward the goal of standardizing the manner in which individuals think about concerning sexual behavior across a school district. Although you may choose to adopt aspects of this document in ways that suit the needs of your district, it is recommended that you develop the tool you use via a multi-agency strategy because the document will better reflect the needs of your district and agency buy-in will be improved.

The following is a page-by-page discussion of the construction of the Level 1 protocol.

Page 1: The team decided to put the outcome page of the Level 1 meeting on the first page of the document as a means of protecting the contents of the document itself. The idea being that an individual could immediately determine the outcome without flipping through the document itself, which, quite obviously, contains very personal information.

Page 2: This page contains a visual flowchart that specifies the steps and considerations in conducting a Level 1 protocol.

Page 3: This page contains the disclaimer, which should be read at the start of every Level 1 meeting. It also has a brief description of who should attend a Level 1. Following this, the Level 1 protocol begins with a precaution regarding imminent danger as well as a collection of relevant demographic information.

Pages 4–7: These pages contain the questions that are addressed during the Level 1. Please note that after every question there is a rationale for the question. Additionally, following this rationale are suggestions regarding specific supervision strategies contained on pages 10 and 11 that might help address the concern posed by the question.

Page 7: This page contains a sexual behavior continuum designed to serve as a guide regarding the severity of specific sexual behaviors. This continuum also acts as a data collection device. At the bottom of page 7 there is some guidance regarding when to request a Level 2 Response.

Page 8: This page is where the Level 1 team documents their disposition of the case and signs off. Once this is completed, the team marks the case disposition on the first page of the Level 1 protocol.

Page 9: This page describes the theoretical model employed by Salem-Keizer in their consideration of risk. The limitations of this model with regard to sexually concerning behavior is discussed in the chapter on Supervision.

Pages 10–11: These pages detail various supervision options that a district might employ or recommend. Bolded items are typically included in most supervision plans. At the bottom of page 11 is an area where the administrator denotes when he or she intends to review the status of the supervision plan.

Page 12: This page details the process for dispatching a Level 2 consultation and gathers additional relevant information.

Page 13: This page collects the signatures of the Level 1 team and provides information regarding where to send copies of the Level 1 protocol. Team signatures are collected regardless of the disposition of the case.

SALEM KEIZER SCHOOL DISTRICT
SEXUAL INCIDENT RESPONSE SYSTEM
~ LEVEL 1 PROTOCOL ~
(EDITION 2011)

LEVEL 1 OUTCOME
(To be completed at the end of the Level 1 Investigation)

Disposition   **Date**   **Responsible Party**

Referred to Law Enforcement

Dismissed

Developed Supervision Plan

Referred to Level 2

Other

Notes:

- This system is designed to examine sexual incidents that include concerning/inappropriate sexual behavior. It is not designed for use with students who are suicidal, engaging in threatening/violent behavior or who are setting fires, unless they are doing so as part of a sexual act. (If a suicide screening, threat assessment screening or fire-setting screening is needed, please consult the Salem-Keizer counseling website or call support services at 503.399-3101).

- Consult the flow chart below to determine the course of screening. If a Level 1 Incident Assessment is indicated, proceed with the attached Protocol and step-by-step instructions.

SALEM•KEIZER
PUBLIC SCHOOLS

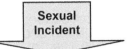

Sexual Incident

UPON DISCOVERY OF THE INCIDENT, THE SCHOOL RESOURCE OFFICER SHOULD BE INFORMED. IF THE EVENT IS FOUND TO BE ILLEGAL, REPORT TO LEVEL OFFICES, AND FOLLOW DISTRICT PROTOCOL GUIDELINES.

Level 1 to be considered by
Administrator & Counselor

Guidelines for consideration of Level 1 (any of the following):

1. Sexual incident occurs at school.
2. School staff is informed about concerning sexual behavior occurring in school or community.
3. Sexual behavior is causing disruption to school activity.
4. There is a history of sexually inappropriate behavior.
5. Staff, parent, or students perceive the sexual incident as unusual, odd, or inappropriate.
6. Administrator is unable to assert that the concern is unfounded.

Unfounded Concern

Level 1 Protocol completed by Site Team

Steps 1-3:
Demographics and screening.

Step 4:
Use supervision strategies to address concerns. Determine if Level 2 is needed by using suggested criteria.

Step 5: (After completing Level 1) if Level 2 is needed call Wilson Kenney at (503) 689-5709 to schedule.

Step 6:
Sign and Fax a copy of the Level 1 AND incident report to Security Department and appropriate Level Office.

- IMPORTANT -
Maintain two copies of the Level 1: One in a letter-size manila envelope marked "Confidential" placed in the student's regular academic or cumulative file and a second copy in a working file in the administrator's (case manager's) office. Then update SASI to note the presence of a Confidential Record.

SALEM•KEIZER
PUBLIC SCHOOLS

THIS PROTOCOL IS ONLY TO BE USED BY STAFF WHO HAVE BEEN TRAINED
THROUGH THE LEVEL 1 SCREENING PROCESS. READ AT THE START OF EVERY LEVEL 1 MEETING.
The results of this survey do not predict or diagnose sexual deviance, nor are they designed to assess an individual's or group's risk of harm to others. This survey is not a checklist that can be quantified. It is a guide designed to assist Level 1 teams in making a determination regarding whether the sexual incident in question is normative or non-normative and to assist the school staff in the development of a management plan. This guide is not intended to serve as an investigation of potential danger and should not be employed for the purpose of identifying circumstances and variables that may increase risk for potential sexual misconduct. Furthermore as additional information about a sexual incident is revealed, so may perceptions about the seriousness of the incident change. If you are reviewing this survey at a date after the assessment completion, do so while being mindful of supervision, intervention, and the passage of time.

Complete the following survey through the Site Team Investigation using the noted step-by-step instructions.
The Site Team is composed of the following:

- Administrator (Discipline AP or Principal)
- Counselor
- School Resource Officer (as appropriate)
- Educators or other people who know the student / students

- Parents, if time and circumstances allow / Case Manager if adjudicated or ward of the Court. If parents are unable to attend, complete the Parent Questionnaire through interview.
- Campus Monitor if possible.

Many cases can be managed through a Level 1 Screening with appropriate interventions. The screening usually takes from 20 to 45 minutes and is a way of documenting concerns and management strategies. It is also a way to determine if there is a need to request a more extensive Level 2 Assessment by staff that specializes in Sexual Misconduct investigation (Step 4). If consultation is needed regarding the Level 1 or Level 2 process, please call or email Dr. Wilson Kenney at Student Services (503) 399-3101 or cell (503) 689-5709.

LEVEL 1 SCREENING

STEP 1: MAKE SURE ALL STUDENTS / STAFF ARE SAFE

☐ If necessary take appropriate precautions such as detaining the student and restricting access to coats, backpacks, lockers, etc.

IF *IMMINENT* DANGER EXISTS CALL LAW ENFORCEMENT, LEVEL OFFICE, AND FOLLOW THE DISTRICT SAFETY GUIDELINES.

☐ Notification to parent / guardian of identified targeted student(s) as outlined in district policy.

STEP 2: COMPLETE THE FOLLOWING INFORMATION:

☐ The parent / guardian has been notified that this screening is being done.
☐ The parent / guardian **has not** been notified of this meeting because: _____

☐ Parent questionnaire completed if parent cannot attend (see Sexual Incident Response System Guide).
☐ Parents discouraged from participating by legal counsel.

SCHOOL: _____ SCHOOL PHONE #: _____ TODAY'S DATE: _____

ADMINISTRATOR / CASE MANAGER: _____ DATE OF INCIDENT: _____

STUDENT NAME: _____ STUDENT #: _____ DOB: _____ AGE: ____ GRADE:___

☐ COPY OF DISTRICT INCIDENT REPORT IS ATTACHED.

STEP 3: SCREENING – DISCUSS, INVESTIGATE, AND DOCUMENT

Each question is a prompt for exploration of the nature of the sexual incident. Please note concerns by each item or under other concerns **Review the questions below as an outline for a guided conversation investigating the nature of the sexual incident in question.**

Was a report filed with SRO? ☐ No ☐ Yes
☐ Not applicable (historical incident / previous police contact / no current legal concern)

Was event determined to be illegal by the SRO investigation? ☐ No ☐ Yes ☐ Not applicable

Describe details of sexual incident: _____
_____
_____
_____
_____

PEER TO PEER

1. Are the individuals involved in the sexual incident roughly equivalent in regard to development, cognitive capacity, physical capacity, emotional functioning and coping skills?
☐ No ☐ Yes, if no describe: _____

Note: if individuals differ in regard to age, development or cognitive capacity by three or more years, or if one or more of the individuals involved in the sexual incident are physically incapacitated, the incident in question may represent a concerning power imbalance that warrants further scrutiny.
Consider Supervision Strategies (page 10-11): 18, 20, 50, 52

HISTORICAL DATA
(Gathered via SRO investigation and File Review)

2. Is there a known history of previous sexually inappropriate behavior?
☐ No ☐ Yes, if yes describe: _____
Note: Previous sexually inappropriate behavior suggests that a pattern of maladaptive sexual behavior may be present.

3. Has the student involved in the sexual incident been previously censured, disciplined, or placed on a behavior/safety plan for sexually inappropriate behavior? ☐ No ☐ Yes, if yes describe: ____

Note: Continuing sexually inappropriate behavior in response to censure may suggest a more serious concern regarding sexual misconduct that may warrant closer scrutiny

4. Is there any evidence that the student has been exposed to inappropriate sexual content or behavior?
☐ No ☐ Yes, if yes describe: _____
Note: Research suggests that developmentally premature or inappropriate exposure may play a role in the development of concerning sexual behavior.
Consider Supervision Strategies (page 10-11): 18, 20, 38, 40, 43, 44, 50, 52, 58

INCIDENT DETAILS

SALEM•KEIZER
PUBLIC SCHOOLS

5. Do all parties involved in the sexual incident (when spoken to separately) agree upon the details of the incident?
☐ No   ☐ Yes, if no describe: _____

_____
Note: disagreement may reflect dishonesty and the need of one of the members to conceal the degree to which they instigated the sexual incident or attempted to hide its discovery.

6. Were coercion, violence, threats, force, manipulation, gifts, and/or privileges used by one or more parties as a strategy to facilitate compliance with the sexual incident or maintain secrecy?
☐ No   ☐ Yes, if yes describe: _____

_____
Note: coercion indicates that at least one of the parties involved in the sexual incident put undue pressure on at least one of the other parties, suggesting that further scrutiny is warranted. Pay particularly close attention to any attempt/effort made by any party to maintain secrecy regarding the incident as this speaks to the degree to which the individual had knowledge that the sexual incident was inappropriate.
Consider Supervision Strategies (page 10-11): 6, 40, 43, 49, 50, 51, 52

7. Was the sexual behavior consistent with developmentally normative/common sexual conduct?
☐ No   ☐ Yes, if no describe: _____

_____
Note: developmentally atypical sexual behavior may suggest pathological sexual development that warrants further scrutiny.
Consider Supervision Strategies (page 10-11): 40, 43, 50, 52, 58

8. Did the sexual incident cause physical or emotional pain or discomfort to any of the involved parties?
☐ No   ☐ Yes, if yes describe: _____

_____
Note: sexual behavior that causes emotional, physical pain and/or psychological distress to others suggests that the event in question was harmful and should be examined with further scrutiny.
Consider Supervision Strategies (page 10-11): 40, 50, 52

9. What does the student indicate was the motive for the sexual behavior (how do they explain it)?
Describe: _____

_____
Note: Poor insight, deceptiveness, lack of empathy and minimization may suggest the need for intervention is higher than when these areas are not compromised.
Consider Supervision Strategies (page 10-11): 40, 50, 52

10. Was there an obvious imbalance in power (difference in physical strength or access to

opportunity/resources) among the individuals involved in the sexual incident?

☐ No   ☐ Yes, if yes describe: _____

_____

Note: an imbalance of power may suggest that coercion played a role in the sexual incident.
Consider Supervision Strategies (page 10-11): 6, 40, 43, 49, 50, 51, 52

11. Was a weapon present during the sexual incident?

☐ No   ☐ Yes, if yes describe: _____

_____

Note: a weapon refers to any object that may be used to threaten physical or emotional safety (i.e. not limited to conventional weapons such as knives or firearms). The mere presence of a weapon, whether employed in a threatening manner or not, may suggest that coercion was employed.
Consider Supervision Strategies (page 10-11): 6, 40, 43, 49, 50, 51, 52

12. Did grooming occur in the context of the sexual incident (refer to the Grooming Behaviors?

☐ No   ☐ Yes, if yes describe: _____

_____

Note: grooming suggests that strong sexual intent and manipulation played a role in the sexual incident which may require further scrutiny.
Consider Supervision Strategies (page 10-11): 40, 50, 52

13. Did staff, parents or others voice a strong visceral response regarding the sexual incident?

☐ No   ☐ Yes, if yes describe: _____

_____

Note: a strong visceral response suggests that individuals have a serious concern that is difficult to verbalize. Further scrutiny of the incident is recommended.

OTHER CONCERNS

Enuretic/Encopretic? ☐ No ☐ Yes Past / Present *Consider Supervision Strategies: 40, 49*	**Impulsive?** ☐ No ☐ Yes *Consider Supervision Strategies: 13, 15*
Harms Animals? ☐ No ☐ Yes Past / Present *Consider Supervision Strategies: 40, 49*	**Opportunistically Vigilant?** ☐ No ☐ Yes *Consider Supervision Strategies: 15, 17, 20, 21,*
Planful? ☐ No ☐ Yes *Consider Supervision Strategies: 30, 40, 49*	

Threatening Behavior

Suicidal Ideation? ☐ No ☐ Yes Past / Present *Consider Supervision Strategies: 4, 5, 40, 49*	☐ Refer for Suicide Risk Assessment
Targeted Threat? ☐ No ☐ Yes Past / Present *Consider Supervision Strategies: 6, 40, 49*	☐ Refer for Student Threat Assessment
Firesetting? ☐ No ☐ Yes Past / Present *Consider Supervision Strategies: 7, 40, 49*	☐ Refer for Firesetting Assessment

Other Concerns (DHS involvement, multiple foster placements, mental health concerns, health concerns, important historical factors, exposure to abuse/neglect, current mood, sleep routine,

SALEM•KEIZER
PUBLIC SCHOOLS

appetite, medication, familial history of sexual misconduct, etc.):

_____
_____
_____
_____
_____

Based upon the aforementioned information:
Circle the nature of the sexual incident of concern
Sexual Behavior Continuum (Consider AGE, FORCE and CONTEXT as a factor)

Lower Concern ⟵   ⟶ Higher Concern

| Flirting/Sexual Harassment | Public kissing/hugging | Peeping | Sexual talk/drawing/gesturing | Rubbing pubic area against object | Public masturbation | Exposing sexual parts | Over the clothes sexual touching | Rubbing pubic area against person | Under the clothes non-penetrative sexual touching | Penetrative sexual touching | Penetrative sex |

CONSIDER REQUESTING A <u>LEVEL 2 SEXUAL INCIDENT RESPONSE</u> IF:

1. The sexual incident appears non-normative and/or severe with regard to intensity,
   and / or
2. You have clear concerns but are unable to confidently answer questions on this protocol,
   and / or
3. You have confidently answered the questions on this protocol and have safety concerns that are beyond your Site Team's ability to supervise and secure within the building,
   and / or
4. You have exhausted your building resources and would like to explore community support to assist you with supervision.
   and/or

   See Step 5 for Level 2 Sexual Incident Response referral process.

LEVEL 1 OUTCOME

7

(To be completed at the end of the Level 1 Investigation)		
Disposition	**Date**	**Responsible Party**
☐ Refer to Law Enforcement		
☐ Dismiss		
☐ Develop Supervision Plan		
☐ Refer to Level 2		
Notification & Release	**Date**	**Responsible Party**
☐ DHS		
☐ Law Enforcement		
☐ Private Therapist		
☐ Liberty House		
☐ Juvenile Justice		

Notes:_____

_____

Participants:

Administrator	Other:
Counselor	Other:
SRO	Other:

STEP 4: DEVELOP A SUPERVISION PLAN TO ADDRESS CONCERNS
(Including aggravating factors) IDENTIFIED THROUGH STEP 3.

SALEM•KEIZER
PUBLIC SCHOOLS

Opportunity
Method

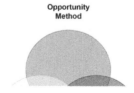

8

Sexual Incidents occur at the intersection of Opportunity, Access and Intent.
In supervision planning, one should be mindful of the degree to which our strategies limit
Access and Opportunity, and consider the nature of the student's Intent.

Perceived Intent:
☐ Engage in concerning sexual behavior
☐ Unknown
☐ Other (Specify):_____

Target (mark all that apply):
☐ Younger children (specify age):_____   ☐ Males
☐ Peers   ☐ Females
☐ Compromised Peers (specify):_____   ☐ Other:_____
☐ Adults

Opportunities (mark all that apply):
☐ Transitions/Lining-up   ☐ Classroom
☐ Recess/Lunch/Assemblies   ☐ Walking Home
☐ Bathroom   ☐ Community
☐ Technology use   ☐ Home
☐ Bus   ☐ Other:_____
☐ Aftercare

SALEM•KEIZER
PUBLIC SCHOOLS

9

STEP 4 *Continued*

RECOMMENDED INTERVENTIONS (CHECK ☒ IF IMPLEMENTED):
Bolded Items are typically included in most supervision plans

Individual Options:
1. ☐ Intended victim warned – parent/guardian notified (see Notification form)
2. ☐ Protective Response initiated by Security Department
3. ☐ **Individual Accountability Plan**
   Detail Expectations of Plan (e.g. Hands to work, No sexual talk, etc.): _____
   _____

4. ☐ Suicide Assessment initiated on _____ (use District Suicide Protocol)
                           date
5. ☐ No harm contract
6. ☐ Threat Assessment initiated on _____ (use District Threat Assessment Protocol)
                           date
7. ☐ Firesetter Assessment initiated on _____ (use District Firesetter Assessment Protocol)
                           date
8. ☐ Other: _____

School Options:
9. ☐ Bus Supervision, Specify:_____

10. ☐ Student Escorted from Transport to School Office, and from Classroom to Transport by:_____

11. ☐ Student Escorted from School Office to Classroom and back by Adult, Specify:_____
12. ☐ **Line-of-Sight Supervision (Zone)**
13. ☐ Arms-Reach Supervision (One-on-one)
14. ☐ Supervised Lunch/Breaks/Recess/Assembly
15. ☐ Special Classroom Seating Assignment (to increase supervision)
16. ☐ No After-School Activities
17. ☐ Supervised After-School Activities (Specify in Safety Plan)
18. ☐ Academic Restrictions (e.g. not involved in childcare courses, mentoring younger students, technology)
   Specify:_____
19. ☐ No Access to Technology
20. ☐ Supervised Access to Technology
21. ☐ Bathroom Plan, Specify: _____
22. ☐ Review educational plan
23. ☐ Social Work Services
24. ☐ Travel card and time accountability
25. ☐ Social skills building programs
26. ☐ Increase supervision in following settings in the following ways: _____
27. ☐ Modifications of daily schedule ☐ Late arrival / early dismissal
28. ☐ **Alert staff on need-to-know basis, Specify staff:**
   ☐ **All supervisory staff** ☐ **Teacher only** ☐ **Teacher and I.A.'s only** ☐ **SRO** ☐ **Office staff**
   Staff member responsible for alerting staff and teachers:_____
29. ☐ Random Check of backpack, locker, pocket, purse, etc. by:
   ☐ Administrator ☐ CDS / Counselor ☐ SRO ☐ Other_____
30. ☐ Assign identified staff to build trusting relationship through check-in or mentorship:
   ☐ Administrator ☐ Mentor ☐ CDS/ Counselor ☐ School Resource Officer ☐ Teacher ☐ Other: _____
31. ☐ Other interventions or supervision strategies that will likely decrease the possibility of a future sexual incident
   Describe: _____

SALEM•KEIZER
PUBLIC SCHOOLS

STEP 4 *Continued*

(NOTE: If student is on IEP/504 plan, any change in placement or Special Ed services must be done through Special Education Team process or 504 team process.)

32. ☐ Referral to appropriate school team to consider alternative placement
33. ☐ Home supervision pending further assessment
34. ☐ Increased supervision in the following settings: _____
35. ☐ Referral to appropriate Special Ed. Team to consider Psycho Educational Evaluation / Special Education Assessment or Behavior Team Referral. **(NOTE: Must be done through Special Education Team Process.)**

☐ Other: _____

_____

Family / Home Options:

Guardians encouraged to:

36. ☐ No Access to Technology
37. ☐ Supervised Access to Technology
38. ☐ Line-of-Sight Supervision
39. ☐ Safety Proof home
40. ☐ Review & pursue crisis/mental health services
41. ☐ **Provide detailed information regarding safety concerns to care providers when leaving child in care of others**
42. ☐ Increase supervision (specify):_____
_____

43. ☐ Guardian discouraged from allowing sleepovers
44. ☐ Guardian provided list of treatment providers
45. ☐ **Guardian provided list of concerning / grooming behaviors**
46. ☐ **Guardian discouraged from allowing contact between students involved in sexual incident**
47. ☐ Other: _____
_____

Encouraged Community Options:

_____ encouraged to pursue:
(community organization)

48. ☐ Referral to YST
49. ☐ Mental Health evaluation
50. ☐ Psychosexual evaluation
51. ☐ Anger management programs
52. ☐ Sexual Misconduct / Interpersonal Boundaries programs
53. ☐ Alcohol / Drug evaluation

54. ☐ Parenting Programs
55. ☐ Mentoring programs
56. ☐ Notify Probation / Parole officer
57. ☐ Faith Based Community Programs
58. ☐ Liberty House
59. ☐ Mid-Valley Women's Crisis Center

Other Options: _____

_____

_____

_____

Review:

☐ Administrator will review the status of this plan and revise as needed on: _____
(date)

SALEM•KEIZER
PUBLIC SCHOOLS

STEP 5: After completion of the Level 1 Screening, and if the Site Team has determined that a Level 2 Meeting is needed,

Immediately contact **Wilson Kenney** at **(503) 689-5709** to begin the process and

Fax a copy of the Level 1 to **Rhonda Stueve** at **(503) 375-7815**.

Please provide Dispatch with the information requested below so a complete Level 2 team can be assembled in a timely manner.

If a Level 2 Response is not requested, move to Step 6 to complete the protocol.

NOTE:
While awaiting the Level 2 Response, use the student supervision plan (Step 4) to manage the situation and document interim steps taken by Site Team.

INFORMATION NEEDED FOR DISPATCHING A LEVEL 2

1. **Is student adjudicated?** ☐ Yes ☐ No
   If yes – Name of Probation Officer _____ Phone #:_____

2. **A Ward of the Court or other supervision?** ☐ Yes ☐ No
   If yes – Name of Caseworker _____ Phone#: _____

3. **Other agencies or individuals involved with the student (therapists, doctors, etc.) that should be included with the parent's permission?** ☐ Yes ☐ No
   If yes, is there signed consent for exchange of information? ☐ Yes ☐ No
   If yes, please list agencies and individuals: _____ Phone: _____
   _____ Phone: _____
   _____ Phone: _____

4. **Special Ed. Or 504 involvement, disability codes and current placement?** ☐ Yes ☐ No
   If yes, details:_____

5. **Is student in self-contained classroom?** ☐ Yes ☐ No

6. **Was parent or guardian present at Level 1 survey:** ☐ Yes ☐ No

7. **Are parents supportive, constructive and available to attend Level 2?** ☐ Yes ☐ No
   If yes, what is their contact information: Home Phone:_____Cell Phone:_____

8. **Other information Level 2 team will need for assessment:** _____

_____

_____

SALEM•KEIZER
PUBLIC SCHOOLS

STEP 6:
Sign, send, file and begin supervision as planned.

1. Sign the Protocol
2. Fax a copy of the Level 1 Protocol to Rhonda Stueve (503) 375-7815

3. Fax a copy of the Level 1 Protocol to the *Appropriate* Level Office:
   Elementary Education: (503) 375-7804
   Secondary Education (503) 375-7817

4. Maintain two copies of the Level 1.
   One in a letter-size manila envelope marked "Confidential Record" placed in the student's regular academic or cumulative file and *a second* copy in a working file in the Administrator's (case manager's) office.

5. Then update SASI to note the presence of a Confidential Record.

Team Signatures:

_____			_____	
Administrator, Plan Supervisor	Date		Counselor	Date
_____			_____	
School Resource Officer	Date		Other	Date
_____			_____	
Parent	Date		Other	Date
_____			_____	
Other	Date		Other	Date
_____			_____	
Other	Date		Other	Date

Developed by Wilson Kenney, Ph.D. at Salem-Keizer Public Schools using the following information: VanDreal, <u>Salem-Keizer School District Threat Assessment Response System</u>; Friedrich, Fisher, Broughton, Houston and Shafran; Barbaree and Marshall, <u>The Juvenile Sex Offender</u>; <u>Normative Sexual Behavior in Children: A Contemporary Sample</u>; <u>NCSBY Fact Sheet</u>; Kaeser, <u>Towards a Better Understanding of Children's Sexual Behavior</u>; Elliot, <u>Grooming</u>; Stewart, <u>Victim Grooming: Protect your Child from Sexual Predators</u>; Anderson, <u>Continuum of Sexual Behavior</u>; Pynchon and Borum, <u>Assessing Threats of Targeted Group Violence: Contributions from Social Psychology</u>; Reddy, Borum, Berlun, Vossekuil, Fein, and Modzeleski, <u>Evaluating Risk for Targeted Violence in Schools: Comparing Risk Assessment, Threat Assessment, and Other Approaches</u>; O'Toole, <u>The School Shooter: A Threat Assessment Perspective</u>; Fein, Vossekuil and Holden, <u>Threat Assessment: An Approach to Prevent Targeted Violence</u>; Meloy, <u>Violence Risk and Threat Assessment</u>, Specialized Training Services Publication; De Becker, <u>The Gift of Fear</u>; Vossekuil, Pollack, Bourne, Modzekski, Reddy, and Fein, <u>Threat Assessment in Schools, A Guide to Managing Threatening Situations and to Creating Safe School Climates.</u>

SALEM•KEIZER
PUBLIC SCHOOLS

Appendix B

Questionnaires

In some cases, it is important that you be able to gather information from individuals who either cannot or will not attend the Level 1 meeting. In order to plan for such an event, a Teacher Questionnaire and Parent Questionnaire are included. It is recommended that these questionnaires be completed via interview rather than simply handed to the teacher or parent to fill out, because when parents or teachers are left to fill them out independently, they generally come back with very little information.

Additionally, you will note that at the end of each question there are a set of numbers in parentheses. These numbers refer to the question/s on the Level 1 protocol that is/are addressed by the question on the questionnaire and are included here to aid you in referencing the Level 1 protocol.

Appendix B

Salem Keizer School District
Sexual Incident Response and Management System
Parent Questionnaire - Level 1

Step 1: Directions for Case Manager:

This questionnaire is only to be completed by a school counselor or administrator as a supplement to the Level 1 Screening Protocol (by phone or in person) if a parent/guardian does not attend the Level 1 Screening. Address the following questions through an interview or conversation with open-ended inquiry. Do NOT ask the guardian to read and complete the questions by themselves.

Although a parent/guardian can provide crucial information regarding a situation, do not delay the Level 1 Screening if the parent is not available, is unwilling, or if the Site Team determines that the parent should not be included at this time.

The following is an examination of current circumstances and as these circumstances change or additional information is uncovered, so too do the impressions about the sexual incident in question; therefore, review the following questions while being mindful of supervision, intervention and the passage of time. Each question is a prompt for exploration of circumstances surrounding the sexual incident in question.

Student's Name: _____ Date: _____

Administrator / Case Manager's Name: _____

Parent / Guardian's Name: _____

Person completing the questionnaire: _____

Contact parent / guardian and describe threat, dangerous situation or violent action that has brought this student to your attention. Explain our obligation and responsibility to investigate and assess situation that may be dangerous for the student, other students, and/or staff.

Step 2: Ask the following questions through conversation or direct inquiry.

The numbers in parenthesis at the end of each question refer to the corresponding Level 1 Protocol questions that are to be addressed in accordance with the information collected in this questionnaire.

1. Does the student have any developmental/cognitive problems or remarkable physical limitations? (1)

2. Does the student have any history of sexually concerning behavior? (2, 3)

SALEM•KEIZER
PUBLIC SCHOOLS

Page 1

3. Has the student ever been charged with or found guilty of sexual misbehavior? (2, 3)

4. Has the student ever been disciplined or censured informally, by parents, for inappropriate sexual behavior? If so, how did the censure impact his/her behavior? (3)

5. Has the student been exposed to inappropriate sexual content or behavior? (4)

6. Does the student have a history of using coercion (violence, threats, force, manipulation, gifts privileges) to get needs/desires met? (6)

7. To your knowledge, has the student ever engaged in any developmentally unusual sexual behavior, or shown an interest in sexual matters that seemed inappropriate considering the student's development? (7)

8. Does the student have a history of causing harm to others, or bullying? (6, 10)

9. Does the student have access to weapons? (11)

10. Has the student ever employed a weapon to threaten others or get his/her way? (11)

SALEM•KEIZER
PUBLIC SCHOOLS

Page 2

Appendix C

Systems Guide and Flowcharts

The Systems Guide is a brief two-page summary of the sexual incident response process from the moment an incident is discovered until the point at which the case is resolved.

The Systems Flow Chart is a visual representation of the sexual incident response process.

The Level 2 Referral and Guidelines Flowchart provides a visual representation and decision-making matrix for the purpose of helping Level 1 teams make a decision about whether or not to seek consultation from the Level 2 Team.

The Flow Chart—Level 2 is a visual representation of the process that occurs once a Level 2 consultation is requested.

SALEM KEIZER SCHOOL DISTRICT
SEXUAL INCIDENT RESPONSE AND MANAGEMENT SYSTEM
SYSTEMS GUIDE

THE INCIDENT

A. Implied sexual threat (e.g. harassment, sexual bullying) or sexual act occurs (student(s) engaged sexual activity or making sexual threats directed at others.) ***NOTE:*** System is NOT to be used for students who are suicidal, acting out violently, or setting fires, unless they are doing so as a sexual act.

B. **If the sexual incident is thought to be illegal, and not simply a violation of school policy, notify Law Enforcement, appropriate Level Office, and Security Department. Initiate a protective response using district guidelines.**

NEED FOR LEVEL 1

A. The Level 1 Screening is initiated by the administrator with consultation from another member of the Site Team. The Site Team is comprised of administrators, school counselors and school resource officers. (***See Systems Flow Chart***.)

B. The Level 1 Protocol is recommended for investigation and documentation of concerns about the sexual incident and is designed to enable the Level 1 team to make a judgment regarding the developmental normativeness of the sexual incident. A direct sexual threat (expressed or acted out), or sexual act does not have to be clearly indicated in order to proceed with a Level 1 Screening. Site Teams are encouraged to use the Level 1 Screening to address concerns and document their review of potential danger or safety issues, even if dismissed as minor or unlikely. (The Level 1 Screening process can be used as a reasonably short (20-30 minute's) review or a more extensive and lengthy screening, depending upon the circumstances.)

C. The following are our guidelines for considering a level 1:
   1. A sexual incident has occurred.
   2. Concern about sexual threat and/or sexual misconduct is causing considerable fear or disruption to activity.
   3. Student has not responded to previous censure for inappropriate sexual behavior.
   4. There is a history of concerning sexual misconduct.
   5. Staff, parent, or student express concerns about sexual behavior.
   6. Administrator is unable to determine if a situation poses a risk to school personnel, students or the community.

LEVEL 1

A. Use the following process to conduct a Level 1 Screening:
   1. Schedule screening as soon as Site Team can assemble. Make sure all students/staff are safe. If necessary take appropriate precautions such as detaining the student and restricting access to coats, backpacks, lockers, etc. If imminent danger exists, call law enforcement, level office and follow district safety guidelines.
   2. Include teachers who know student well (especially English, Humanities and Art teachers), Campus Monitor(s), and education case managers if student is on IEP or 504 Plan. The ***Teacher Questionnaire*** is available for education staff to complete if unable to attend meeting.
   3. Also include community agency case managers if student is adjudicated or a Ward of the Court.
   4. The Parent / guardian should be notified that the screening will be taking place and invited to participate if Administrator determines that parents/guardians will be constructive to the screening process. Site Team may elect to complete the screening without notification and/or inclusion of the parent if it is determined that the participation of the parent would compromise the process. Documentation for parental notification is on the Level 1 Screening. The ***Parent Questionnaire*** is available to complete by phone if parent does not attend meeting.
   5. Through team discussion and information gathering, conduct the Level 1 screening using ***Level 1 Protocol.*** The Level 1 Protocol includes demographics, screening questions, supervision strategies to address risk factors, management needs and has recommended criteria for considering further investigation through the Level 2 process.

SALEM•KEIZER
PUBLIC SCHOOLS

LEVEL 1 *Continued~*

6. Use the supervision strategies suggested in Step 4 to address the concerns and aggravating factors identified in Step 3. If the Site Team determines that more investigation is necessary (see step 5-Level 1 Protocol) contact SIRC (Sexual Incident Response Committee) Dispatch at **503.689.5709**. SIRC Dispatch will then schedule the Level 2 Investigation Team. Upon calling SIRC Dispatch, have the information available requested under step 5 of Level 1 Screening Protocol. This will allow Dispatch to schedule the appropriate attendees (Juvenile Probations Officers, State Case Workers, Therapists, etc.) for the Level 2 Assessment.

B. Use the following process to complete the Level 1 process:
1. Sign and Fax a copy of Level 1 and Incident Report to Wilson Kenney at Student Services (503.375.7812) and appropriate Level Office(s).
2. If other student(s) has been identified as a possible targeted victim notify his / her parents/guardians using the ***Notification Log*** *and the* ***Notification Letter*** (notification call is to be done within 12 hours; notification letter within 24 hours. See ORS. 339.250). Then consider completing a ***Plan to Protect Targeted or Victimized Student*** taking into consideration information from the targeted student and his or her parent/guardians.
3. **Maintain two copies of Level 1 Protocol.** One in a letter-size manila envelope marked, ***Confidential Record*** placed in the student's regular academic or cumulative file and a second copy in the administrator's working file (available to counselor/CDS, and SRO). The case is tracked and managed by the school administrator. Schedule follow up dates for review of supervision plan and risk factors as needed. Update SASI to note the presence of a Confidential Record.

LEVEL 2

A Level 2 Investigation is conducted primarily at the school site by an investigative team comprised of a School Psychologist, Mental Health Worker, Law Enforcement Threat Assessment Specialist and other Case Workers as appropriate (such as Juvenile Probation Counselor, Oregon Youth Authority Counselor or and DHS Case Manager). The investigative team represents the Mid-Valley Sexual Incident Response Committee (or SIRC) with membership from the following agencies:

- Salem Keizer School District
- Site Team (Facilitator)
- Willamette ESD
- Marion County Sheriff's Office
- Salem Police Department
- Keizer Police Department

- Marion County Mental Health
- Polk County Mental Health
- Crisis Team
- Marion County Juvenile Dept.
- Polk County Juvenile Dept.
- Oregon Youth Authority

- Court Authority
- Liberty House
- New Solutions
- Marion County D.D. Services
- Department of Human Services

After the investigation is conducted and management strategies are determined, the student's case will be scheduled for further Level 2 review and advisement with the entire Sexual Incident Response Committee noted above. *(**See Level 2 Flow Chart.**)* A member of the Site Team (the administrator in most cases) will also attend the SIRC staffing. SIRC consultation will further advise on risk, management and intervention strategies, community resources and will support school and other agency professionals on the management of dangerous situations.

Once a student is staffed, case management will be done from the school site by the building administrator and reviewed on a schedule determined at the time of the assessment or as needed if situation escalates. Members of SIRC will provide follow up and consultation as circumstances change and/or supervision needs increase. Student may be reviewed and re-assessed at any time upon the request of the Site Team.

A Level 2 Assessment Summary documenting the risk factors and supervision strategies will be written and provided to the Site Team. Place copies of the Level 2 Investigation Summary in the *Confidential Record* noted above and update SASI to note the presence of a Confidential Record.

SALEM•KEIZER
PUBLIC SCHOOLS

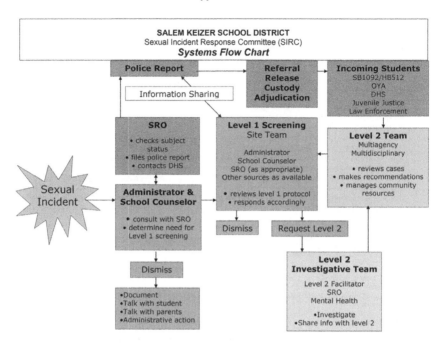

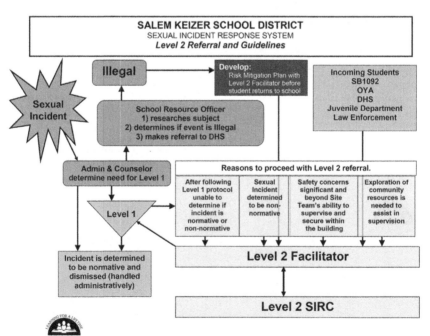

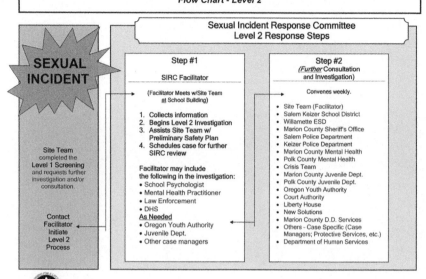

SALEM KEIZER SCHOOL DISTRICT
SEXUAL INCIDENT RESPONSE AND MANAGEMENT SYSTEM
Flow Chart - Level 2

Sexual Incident Response Committee
Level 2 Response Steps

SEXUAL INCIDENT

Site Team completed the **Level 1 Screening** and requests further investigation and/or consultation.

Contact Facilitator Initiate Level 2 Process

Step #1

SIRC Facilitator

(Facilitator Meets w/Site Team at School Building)

1. Collects information
2. Begins Level 2 Investigation
3. Assists Site Team w/ Preliminary Safety Plan
4. Schedules case for further SIRC review

Facilitator may include the following in the investigation:
• School Psychologist
• Mental Health Practitioner
• Law Enforcement
• DHS
As Needed
• Oregon Youth Authority
• Juvenile Dept.
• Other case managers

Step #2
(Further Consultation and Investigation)

Convenes weekly.

• Site Team (Facilitator)
• Salem Keizer School District
• Willamette ESD
• Marion County Sheriff's Office
• Salem Police Department
• Keizer Police Department
• Marion County Mental Health
• Polk County Mental Health
• Crisis Team
• Marion County Juvenile Dept.
• Polk County Juvenile Dept.
• Oregon Youth Authority
• Court Authority
• Liberty House
• New Solutions
• Marion County D.D. Services
• Others - Case Specific (Case Managers; Protective Services, etc.)
• Department of Human Services

SALEM·KEIZER PUBLIC SCHOOLS

Appendix D

Level 2 Inquiry, Level 2 Summary, and Level 2 Letter

The Sexual Incident Inquiry is a data collection tool used by the Level 2 facilitator when responding to a request for a Level 2. After the Level 1 team meeting and before the Level 2 team meeting, the Level 2 facilitator sets up a meeting with the administrator and/or the school counselor requesting the Level 2. During that meeting, the Level 2 facilitator gathers additional information from the referring school about the student for the purpose of sharing this information with the Level 2 team.

The form is referred to as an "inquiry tool" rather than an "investigation tool," which might otherwise suggest this is a form used by law enforcement. Neither is the tool referred to as an "assessment tool," which might suggest that it is an instrument used for psychological assessment.

The Summary of Level 2 inquiry is a tool designed to document the case disposition agreed upon by the Level 2 team. During or directly following the Level 2 meeting, the Level 2 facilitator documents the Level 2 case disposition and recommendations on this form, which is then shared with the referring Level 1 team and placed in the confidential file folder next to the initial Level 1 protocol.

The Level 2 Letter accompanies the Summary of the Level 2 inquiry that is sent out to school administrators.

SEXUAL INCIDENT RESPONSE AND MANAGEMENT SYSTEM
Sexual Incident Inquiry
~ Level 2~

This protocol was developed by Wilson Kenney, School Psychologist, Salem-Keizer School District. It is a structured outline to be used only by professionals trained in SIRC inquiry, mental health/behavioral assessment, and psychoeducational assessment.

Student Name(s):_____Age:___Grade: _____Student Number(s):_____DOB:_____

Today's Date: _____School:_____Administrative Case Manager:_____

Description of the Incident:_____

_____

_____

_____

_____

- ☐ 504 ☐ Spec. Ed ☐ Regular Ed ☐ Adjudication ☐ Ward of State/Court ☐ Foster Care

- Testing information if available:

- Disciplinary action taken:

- Safety planning put in place by school:

SITUATION OR INCIDENT FACTORS:

Targets of Concern
☐ Younger children (specify age):_____   ☐ Males
☐ Peers   ☐ Females
☐ Compromised Peers (specify):_____   ☐ Other:_____
☐ Adults

4/1/10

Sexual Behavior Continuum
Consider AGE, FORCE and CONTEXT as a factor

←━━→

Flirting/Sexual Harassment	Public kissing/hugging	Peeping	Sexual talk/drawing/gesturing	Frotteurism toward an object	Public masturbation	Exposing sexual parts	Over the clothes sexual touching	Frotteurism toward a person	Under the clothes non-penetrative sexual touching	Penetrative sexual touching	Penetrative sex

Details suggesting that the incident was concerning:

☐ Significant difference (>3 years) in regard to:
   ☐ Age
   ☐ Cognitive development
   ☐ Emotional development (coping skills, behavior)
   ☐ Physical capacity
☐ History of sexually inappropriate bx
☐ Previously censured for sexually inappropriate bx
☐ Disagreement regarding details of incident
☐ Evidence of grooming
☐ Strong visceral response among staff/parents
☐ Confusion/Discomfort among involved parties

☐ Attempts at gaining compliance/secrecy:
   ☐ Coercion
   ☐ Violence (or threat of violence)
   ☐ Force
   ☐ Manipulation
   ☐ Gifts/Privileges
☐ Developmentally non-normative incident
☐ Incident caused physical/emotional pain
☐ Confusion about appropriateness of incident
☐ Imbalance of power
☐ Weapon was present

Suggested nature of the of the incident/concern:

Normative		Non-normative	

←━━→

Normative Affection Playful Flirting	Sexually Normative but Mutually Inappropriate Sexual Behavior	Sexually Aggressive & Sexually Non-normative Behavior	Illegal Sexual Behavior

- Preparation/grooming related behavior?

4/1/10

- Other students / people involved (supporting / allowing acting out, ideation, planning)?

  Student Name(s):_____Age:___Grade: _____ (Level 1 or Level 2 assessment complete? Y/N)

  _____   ___   _____ (Level 1 or Level 2 assessment complete? Y/N)

  _____   ___   _____ (Level 1 or Level 2 assessment complete? Y/N)

- Motive?

- Circumstances that might increase risk for sexual misconduct:

- Inhibitors and protective factors (stable living situation, student manages anger well, student has support system, student appears concerned about managing sexual behavior, student recognizes need for support, student recognizes risk factors, student demonstrates willingness to follow safety plan):

Situation/Incident factor concerns are:
☐ **Unremarkable / low**   ☐ **Decreasing**   ☐ **Ongoing**   ☐ **Escalating**

SCHOOL FACTORS

- Academics:

- Attendance:

- Attachment to school:

- Behavioral history:

- Discipline history:

- Educational goals or plan:

- Other School Concerns:

School factor concerns are:
☐ **Unremarkable / low**   ☐ **Decreasing**   ☐ **Ongoing**   ☐ **Escalating**

4/1/10

Appendix D

SOCIAL FACTORS

- Relationships with non-family adults (teachers, community leaders, church, clubs, etc.):

- Interpersonal history at school, home and community (real or perceived):

- Social status

- Peer group (culture, subculture, clique or marginalized clique).

- Role within peer group

- Peers, culture or community endorse unhealthy sexual attitudes?

- Community support level:

Social factor concerns are:
☐ **Unremarkable / low**   ☐ **Decreasing**   ☐ **Ongoing**   ☐ **Escalating**

4/1/10

PERSONAL FACTORS

- Pattern of behavior:

- Personally views sexual behavior as acceptable and normative?

- Emotional coping skills and reserves

- Attitude
  - [ ] self as superior
  - [ ] sees self as a victim
  - [ ] entitled
  - [ ] criminal
  - [ ] narcissistic

  - [ ] has healthy view of personal strengths and weaknesses
  - [ ] sees self as a failure
  - [ ] sees self as inferior, broken or weak
  - [ ] other:_____

- Stress level (real or perceived):

- Concerns
  - [ ] awareness of dysfunctional or troubled situation and wants to change
  - [ ] has awareness but lacks concern or doesn't care
  - [ ] is unaware of dysfunctional or troubled situation

- Trust level:

Sexual Behavior/Attitudes:

- Previously adjudicated for sexual misconduct
  - [ ] >2 previous victims of sexual abuse
  - [ ] previous offense/s suggests planning
  - [ ] previous offense/s involved coercion
  - [ ] penetrative sexual act

  - [ ] previous offense/s involved violence
  - [ ] offended same victim >1
  - [ ] attempt to hide previous sexual misconduct

  Previous victim/s:
  - [ ] male only   [ ] female only   [ ] both   [ ] > 3 year age difference developmentally
  - [ ] interfamilial   [ ] extrafamilial   [ ] stranger

- Previously attended treatment for sexual misconduct
  - [ ] Successfully completed   [ ] Failed to complete   [ ] Maximum benefit

- Past treatment/intervention accessibility and response
  - [ ] accessible   [ ] guarded   [ ] poor response   [ ] resistive   [ ] hostile

4/1/10

Concern	Y	N	Concern	Y	N
Unusual sexual interests/behaviors?			Student understands risk factors?		
Concerns regarding sexual development?			Student is interested in changing behavior?		
Sexually Preoccupied?			Student evidences empathy toward victims?		
Student is concerned about sexual behavior?					
Pornography Use?					

Specify:

- Agitators and Triggers:

Concerning Historical Factors:

Concern	Y	N	Concern	Y	N
Animal abuse?			Central Nervous System damage or TBI?		
Fire-play?			Impulse or inattention problems?		
Property destruction?			Emotional trauma or victim of abuse?		
Drug / alcohol use?			Previous psychiatric treatment?		
Mental Health diagnosis:			Early police contact (prior to age 12)		

Specify:

- Medications:

- Prior arrests:

- Use of a weapon in past (to hurt other human beings)?

Personal factor concerns are:
☐ **Unremarkable / low**   ☐ **Decreasing**   ☐ **Ongoing**   ☐ **Escalating**

FAMILY DYNAMIC FACTORS

- Resides with:

- Siblings?

- Custody?

- Familial history of:
  - [ ] Domestic Violence   [ ] Neglect   [ ] Criminal activity
  - [ ] Mental illness   [ ] Substance abuse   [ ] Previous sanctions for sexual misconduct
  - [ ] Abuse

- Parents /guardians support level:

- Family dynamic and relationships (parental, sibling):

- Parents and or family views regarding sexual behavior?

- Lack of supervision within the household?

- Family is interested in seeking treatment/help for student?

- Family is concerned about students sexual behavior?

- Poor parental control and/or few limits on behavior?

- Computer access within home? Supervised computer access?

- Extended family support level:

Family Dynamic factor concerns are:
[ ] **Unremarkable / low**   [ ] **Decreasing**   [ ] **Ongoing**   [ ] **Escalating**

4/1/10

SALEM•KEIZER
PUBLIC SCHOOLS

Appendix D

SEXUAL INCIDENT RESPONSE AND MANAGEMENT SYSTEM
Summary of Level 2 Inquiry

Today's Date: _____ Date of Incident: _____ School: _____

Student Name(s): _____ Student Number(s): _____

Name of Other Students if Involved: _____

_____

DOB: _____ Age: ____ Grade: ___ Administrative Case Manager: _____

> This summary was generated through the efforts of the sexual incident response system (a set of protocols used by members of the Sexual Incident Response Committee referred to as "SIRC"). The summary: 1) identifies concerns that arose during the case investigation, 2) communicates the case disposition (i.e. interventions, supervision/safety planning, and risk mitigation strategies that were recommended) and 3) identifies the factors that suggest additional risk mitigation planning is warranted. It should be noted that this summary is not a psychosexual report or a prediction of future risk for sexual misconduct, nor is it a foolproof method of assessing an individual's short or long-term risk of harming others sexually. Since it is an examination of current circumstances (and as these circumstances change, so too does the disposition), please review the contents while being mindful of supervision, intervention and the passage of time. For information regarding the Level 1 or Level 2 threat assessment process or the contents of this report, please contact SIRC as represented by J. Wilson Kenney, Salem-Keizer School District (503) 399-3101.

SEXUAL INCIDENT RESPONSE COMMITTEE (SIRC)
The Sexual Incident Response Committee or SIRC is comprised of the following: Salem-Keizer School District, Willamette Educational Services District (WESD), Marion County Sheriff's Office, Salem Police Department, Keizer Police Department, Oregon Judicial Department, Marion County Children's Mental Health, Polk County Children's Mental Health, Marion County Juvenile Dept., Polk County Juvenile Dept., Oregon Youth Authority and Oregon Department of Human Services. SIRC is a consultation team that examines concerns concerning sexual incidents that impact education and assists case managers with the application of resources to manage and decrease the possibility of future sexual misconduct, and support students to develop and employ healthy and safe coping strategies.

REFERRAL

This student was referred for Level 2 threat assessment because:
- [ ] The sexual incident appears non-normative,
- [ ] Staff have clear concerns but are unable to confidently answer questions on this protocol,
- [ ] Staff have confidently answered the questions on this protocol and have safety concerns that are beyond the Site Team's ability to supervise and secure within the building,
- [ ] Staff have exhausted building resources and would like to explore community support to assist with supervision.
- [ ] Other: _____

SALEM•KEIZER
PUBLIC SCHOOLS

INCIDENT/CONCERN

The following is a description of the incident or concern:_____
_____
_____
_____

Context in which the incident occurred and details of the incident:

Place:_____
_____

Structure level:
☐ Low ☐ Moderate ☐ High ☐ Any

Social situation:_____
_____

Target of sexual behavior:	Expression of sexual behavior:	
☐ Females	☐ Sexual talk / drawings	☐ Over the clothes sexual
☐ Males	☐ Sexually aggressive	touching of others
☐ Adults	posturing	☐ Under the clothes sexual
☐ Developmentally	☐ Sexual kissing	touching of others
equivalent peers	☐ Frotteurism (rubbing	☐ Penetrative sex
☐ Developmentally	genitals against	☐ Threatened forcible sex
compromised peers	someone/something)	☐ Forced sex
☐ Younger children: _____	☐ Exposing genitals	☐ other:_____
age range	☐ Public masturbation	_____
☐ other:_____		

☐ Influenced by peer pressure or gang related:
☐ Influenced by drugs and alcohol:
☐ Criminal act:

Details suggesting that the incident was concerning:

☐ Significant difference (>3 years) in regard to:	☐ Attempts at gaining compliance/secrecy:
☐ Age	☐ Coercion
☐ Cognitive development	☐ Violence (or threat of violence)
☐ Emotional development (coping skills, behavior)	☐ Force
☐ Physical capacity	☐ Manipulation
☐ History of sexually inappropriate bx	☐ Gifts/Privileges
☐ Previously censured for sexually inappropriate bx	☐ Developmentally non-normative incident
☐ Disagreement regarding details of incident	☐ Incident caused physical/emotional pain
☐ Evidence of grooming	☐ Confusion about appropriateness of incident
☐ Strong visceral response among staff/parents	☐ Imbalance of power
☐ Confusion/Discomfort among involved parties	☐ Weapon was present

Appendix D

INCIDENT/CONCERN:

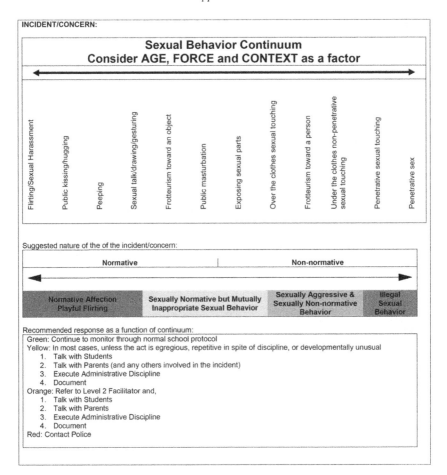

Sexual Behavior Continuum
Consider AGE, FORCE and CONTEXT as a factor

Suggested nature of the of the incident/concern:

Normative	Non-normative

Normative Affection Playful Flirting	Sexually Normative but Mutually Inappropriate Sexual Behavior	Sexually Aggressive & Sexually Non-normative Behavior	Illegal Sexual Behavior

Recommended response as a function of continuum:

Green: Continue to monitor through normal school protocol

Yellow: In most cases, unless the act is egregious, repetitive in spite of discipline, or developmentally unusual
1. Talk with Students
2. Talk with Parents (and any others involved in the incident)
3. Execute Administrative Discipline
4. Document

Orange: Refer to Level 2 Facilitator and,
1. Talk with Students
2. Talk with Parents
3. Execute Administrative Discipline
4. Document

Red: Contact Police

SALEM•KEIZER
PUBLIC SCHOOLS

CASE DISPOSITION & RECOMMENDATIONS

These recommendations were generated through the efforts of the 24-J Sexual Incident Response Committee (SIRC) and are for consideration in the management of sexually concerning incidents and circumstances involving students. SIRC is a consultation team that investigates sexual incidents and assists case managers with the application of resources to manage and decrease the possibility of future sexual misconduct, and support students to develop and employ healthy and safe sexual behavior.

(CHECK ☒ IF RECOMMENDED)

Next Steps:

☐ Case will be staffed by Sexual Incident Response Committee (SIRC).
☐ Administrator will request further assessment if risk circumstances escalate. Call: (503)-399-3101.

☐ Continue with Level 1 Student Supervision Plan
☐ Intended victim warned
☐ Parent / Guardian of targeted student notified

Student Options:

☐ Individual Accountability Plan: No harm contract / Student will self manage: Describe:
☐ Suicide Assessment initiated on _____(use District Suicide Protocol.)
☐ Student Threat Assessment initiated on _____(use STAT Protocol.)
☐ Student Firesetter Assessment initiated on _____(use District Firesetter Protocol.)
☐ Student will identify triggers, agitators and agree to "safe room" or resource of support.
☐ Diversion

School Options:

☐ Protective Response initiated by Security Department
☐ Alert staff and teachers on need-to-know basis
☐ Bus Supervision (Specify in Safety Plan)
☐ Student Escorted from Bus to School Office, and from Classroom to School Bus
☐ Student Escorted to and from School Office by Adult, Specify:_____
☐ Line-of-Sight Supervision
☐ Arms-Reach Supervision
☐ Supervised Lunch/Breaks/Recess/Assembly
☐ Special Classroom Seating Assignment (to increase supervision)
☐ No After-School Activities
☐ Supervised After-School Activities (Specify in Safety Plan)
☐ Academic Restrictions (e.g. not involved in childcare courses, or mentoring younger students)
☐ No Access to Technology
☐ Supervised Access to Technology
☐ Review educational plan
☐ Specialized class / Alternative class or track
☐ Travel card and time accountability
☐ Late arrival / early dismissal
☐ Entry / Exit check with:
☐ Continue to monitor communications and behavior.
☐ Other School option: _____
_____

☐ Social skill building programs
☐ Increase supervision in following settings:
☐ Decrease or eliminate pass time or unsupervised time
☐ Daily ☐ Weekly modification of schedule:
☐ Random search of backpack/purse, locker, pockets, etc. by school personnel:
☐ Assign identified staff to build trusting relationship through check-in or mentorship:
  ☐ Administrator   ☐ Counselor   ☐ Mentor
  ☐ School Resource Officer   ☐ Teacher   ☐ Other:
☐ Provide means by which student may safely report and discuss thoughts or intentions to harm others and receive appropriate intervention.
☐ Identify and further develop activities, relationships or things of value that inhibit possibility of acting out:
☐ Other interventions or supervision strategies that will directly address the triggers and agitators identified through assessment:
☐ School Counselor intervention including:
☐ Refer to PIRS or other school resource:
☐ Consider placement change (administrative transfer, Interim Alternative Educational Setting (IAES), expulsion, etc. as per district policy. (District may unilaterally remove student to IAES, but IEP team decides actual placement if student is receiving specialized instruction. See gray box below.)
☐ Safety planning at site of attendance (home school; SPED placement; Alternative Ed.; IDT.

CASE DISPOSITION & RECOMMENDATIONS

☐ Refer to school special education or 504 team to consider evaluation. If student has IEP or 504 plan refer to special education team or 504 team to consider:
　　☐ Further evaluation
　　☐ Reviewing goals and placement options
　　☐ Referral to alternative educational placement
　　☐ Increasing supervision in the following setting: _____
　　☐ Home supervision pending further assessment or action.

Family / Home Options:

☐ Strategize Safety options / planning
☐ Increase supervision
☐ No Access to Technology
☐ Supervised Access to Technology
☐ Line-of-Sight Supervision
☐ Locked Bedrooms for Family Members

☐ Parents contacted and will provide following supervision / intervention:
☐ Safety proof home
☐ Referral for Domestic Violence intervention
☐ Parent training classes.
☐ Other:

Community Options:

☐ Referral to YST
☐ School referred (STAT) mental health valuation
☐ Anger management programs
☐ Mentoring programs
☐ Notify Probation /Parole officer
☐ Faith Community Programs
☐ Foster Positive Community Activities, interests
☐ Refer to Juvenile Family Support Program

☐ Explore grant money assistance for inhibitors or other needs
☐ Referral to substance abuse intervention with:
☐ Referral to Mental Health agency for mental health evaluation contact:
☐ Review of counseling or therapy options.
☐ Juvenile Dept. supervision and release / safety plan
☐ Other: _____

Other Options:

FACTORS SUGGESTIVE THAT ADDITIONAL RISK MITIGATION PLANNING MAY BE WARRANTED

Context in which future incidents may be more likely to occur:

Place:_____
_____

Structure level:
- ☐ Low   ☐ Moderate   ☐ High   ☐ Any

Social situation:_____
_____

Target of sexual behavior:	Expression of sexual behavior:	

☐ Females
☐ Males
☐ Adults
☐ Developmentally
   equivalent peers
☐ Developmentally
   compromised peers
☐ Younger children: _____
          age range
☐ other:_____
_____
	☐ Sexual talk
	☐ Sexually aggressive
	   posturing
	☐ Sexual kissing
	☐ Frotteurism (rubbing
	   genitals against
	   someone/something)
	☐ Exposing genitals
	☐ Public masturbation
		☐ Over the clothes sexual
		   touching of others
		☐ Under the clothes sexual
		   touching of others
		☐ Penetrative sex
		☐ Threatened forcible sex
		☐ Forced sex
		☐ other:_____
		_____

☐ Influenced by peer pressure or gang related:
☐ Influenced by drugs and alcohol:
☐ Criminal act:

Factors which suggest the need for additional consideration

☐ New allegations ☐ Student violates supervision plan ☐ Student's therapist/supervision officer/guardian suggests the need for additional supervision ☐ Student evidences recent escalation in anger or negative affect ☐ Student evidences sudden change in affect/behavior	☐ Student appears to be socially isolating self ☐ Student appears to be actively grooming other students ☐ Student evidencing interpersonal aggression toward others ☐ Recent change in caregiver or living situation ☐ Sudden change in school performance

SUMMARY

If a student's situation changes please call (503) 510-8924 to schedule a review of this case.

Further information regarding this assessment is available by contacting the Case Manager (Administrator) at the student's school, the Liaison Officer assigned to that school or the Sexual Incident Response Committee (as represented by Wilson Kenney at Salem-Keizer School District, Student Services, (503) 399-3101.)

_____   **Copy of Report to: * Wilson Kenney**
Wilson Kenney, Ph.D.   **   * School Site Team**
School Psychologist

TO: **Administrator (aka: Case Manager)**

FROM: **J. Wilson Kenney, Ph.D.**
               School Psychologist
               Risk Intervention / 24J

Enclosed please find a copy of the Level 2 Inquiry Summary. **Please maintain two copies of this document: one in a Letter-Size Manila Envelope marked "Confidential" placed in the student's regular academic or cumulative file and a second copy in a working file in your office. (Your school counselor / CDS should also have a working copy if involved in the supervision and management plan.)   Then update SASI to note the presence of a Confidential Record.**

In addition, please keep in mind the following regarding the Sexual Incident Response Team Process:

1.   Level 2 Sexual Incident Response Committee (SIRC) functions as a consultation team. We assist with the investigation of sexual incidents and situations that pose a threat to school district students and staff. We also assist with supervision planning strategies and resource exploration.

2.   We do not mandate interventions or predict the future. We do not have the authority to bypass or over-ride any Salem-Keizer School District policy or procedure. (This includes the IEP process for placement in Special Education.)

3.   Final decisions for management, intervention, and supervision are made by the school Site Team. Case management remains with the Site Team at the attending school.

This case will be reviewed as indicated on the attached report; however, if you have concerns or information regarding the risk level or accuracy of information, please call me at (503) 689-5709.

Thank you,

J. Wilson Kenney, Ph.D.
School Psychologist
Salem Keizer Public Schools

SALEM•KEIZER
PUBLIC SCHOOLS

Appendix E

Plan to Protect, Notification Log, and Notification Letter

On occasion you will encounter situations where a student makes a direct sexual threat to another person or where you have cause to believe that a particular student poses a legitimate sexual threat to another person. When this occurs, you will need to inform the targeted individual and you can use the Plan to Protect to help you develop a plan to keep the targeted individual safe.

The Notification Log is used to document that you informed the targeted individual and his or her guardian. Once you complete the form, you should place it in the student record of the targeted individual. If the targeted individual is a staff member or outside individual, you would keep a copy of the notification log in a file in your office.

The Notification Letter is a form letter designed to provide written documentation regarding the notification of threat. In addition to informing the individual about the concerning threatening behavior, this document also serves as a liability measure.

SEXUAL INCIDENT RESPONSE SYSTEM
Plan to Protect Targeted or Victimized Student

Student Name: _____   Today's Date: _____

DOB: _____   Student #: _____   School _____   Date(s) of Incident: _____

INCIDENT

Attached is a copy of the District Incident Report dated _____. The following is the plan to protect (student's name) _____ from harm.

SAFETY CONCERNS

The safety issues of concern are: _____
_____
_____

SUPPORT PLAN

After meeting with: o **Administration** o **CDS/Counselor** o **School Resource Officer** *
* **Guardian/Parent** * **Security** o **Special Education** * **Sexual Incident Response Team** * **Other** _____
_____ the following will be implemented:

o Law Enforcement has been notified.
o The parent/guardian of the above student was notified of this incident on _____ and a follow-up letter was sent to parent/guardian on _____ .
                                                        (date)
* Further examination will be pursued through the Sexual Incident Response Team.

The student will aid in his/her own protection by: _____
_____

The student will receive the following support from the school: _____
_____

The student will receive the following support from the community: _____
_____

The student will receive the following support from home: _____
_____

The student will receive the following support from law enforcement: _____
_____

_____
Administrator, Plan Supervisor, Date:
(Will maintain responsibility until reassigned or modified)

_____
Liaison Officer, Date:

_____
Student, Date:

_____
CDS/Counselor, Date:

_____
Parent/Guardian, Date:

_____
Other, Date:

SALEM•KEIZER
PUBLIC SCHOOLS

SEXUAL INCIDENT RESPONSE AND MANAGEMENT SYSTEM
Notification Log
(Use as documentation for notification to legal guardians
of threatened or victimized students – See District Policy.)

☐ An interpreter was used for non-English communication
☐ Attached Copy of District Incident Report

School: _____ Student Name:_____ Student #:_____

Date /Time of Incident: _____ Name of Administrator completing this Form:_____

Parent/Guardian Name: _____	Home #:_____	Work #:_____
Parent/Guardian Name: _____	Home #:_____	Work #:_____
**#1 Emergency Name:_____	Home #:_____	Work #:_____
**#2 Emergency Name:_____	Home #:_____	Work #:_____

**NO INFORMATION REGARDING INCIDENT SHOULD BE GIVEN TO THE EMERGENCY CONTACT PERSON – ONLY PARENT/GUARDIAN.

DOCUMENT CONTACT OR ATTEMPTS TO CONTACT IN LOG BELOW

Name	Number Used	Attempted Date and Time	Message Left

NOTIFICATION CHECK-LIST

❑ Described incident to parent/guardian – parent/guardian's comments (attach additional sheet if necessary):
_____
_____

❑ Informed the parent/guardian that Salem-Keizer School personnel, law enforcement, and other agencies as necessary are investigating the validity of this sexual incident.

❑ Described to parent/guardian any immediate safety measures that have been taken - parent/guardian's comments (attach additional comment sheet if necessary): _____
_____

❑ Notified parent/guardian that a follow-up letter to this conversation will be arriving within a couple of days.

❑ Identified myself as the contact person regarding the school's investigation of this incident and provided the name of the School Resource Officer for the Law Enforcement portion of the investigation (provided officers contact information.)

❑ Notified parent/guardian of meeting scheduled on _____ to develop a Plan to Protect their student from harm.
                                                                      (date)

SALEM•KEIZER
PUBLIC SCHOOLS

SEXUAL INCIDENT RESPONSE SYSTEM

Notification Letter
**(Use as written communication to legal guardians
of threatened or victimized students - See District Policy.)**

Certified mail is recommended

DATE

ADDRESS OF PARENT / GUARDIAN

Dear *Parent/Guardian:*

This letter is a follow-up to our phone conversation of (*date of phone call*). To further ensure the safety of all our students, the Oregon Revised Statutes requires written notification to the parent of a student whom may be at risk for potential harm.

This matter has been referred to the (*police agency*). The contact officer will be the School Resource Officer (*name of officer*) who may be reached at (*phone number*) for information regarding the law enforcement investigation.

The validity of this threat will be investigated by a multi-disciplinary team, which will include law enforcement, school administration and guidance counseling, as well as other disciplines and community agencies as needed. This team is currently assessing risk and implementing safety measures for your student. If you have any further questions, I am the contact person for this team and you may call me at the above number.

Sincerely,

ADMINISTRATOR

SALEM•KEIZER
PUBLIC SCHOOLS

Appendix F
Other Important Forms

The Glossary of Forms and Flow Charts is a brief document that provides a list of all the documents related to the leveled threat assessment process and short summaries regarding the use of each of these tools.

The Glossary of Terms and References provides a list of commonly used terms in schools, threat assessment and sexual misconduct literature for the purpose of helping individuals understand jargon.

The Memorandum of Agreement is a legal document that enables individuals from different agencies to openly discuss cases in the context of the Level 2 team meeting.

The Sign-In Sheet is used during the Level 2 meetings to document which individuals were present for each case that was discussed.

Each member of the Level 2 team signs the confidentiality agreement at the first Level 2 meeting they attend. Generally speaking, the Level 2 facilitator keeps track of the confidentiality agreements and makes sure that all new members sign one at their first Level 2 meeting.

SIRC GLOSSARY OF FORMS AND FLOW CHARTS

District Incident Report: Documents any incident that has occurred and what action was taken, including initiating a Threat Assessment.

Guide: A written outline noting the sequential process steps of the entire student threat assessment system.

Confidential Record: Record (manila envelope) located within students cumulative file. Sometimes marked "Confidential Record," this file may contain copies of threat assessments, suicide risk assessments, restraining orders, and other documentation that is not considered part of the education record. The Confidential Record may be accessed by school administrators, counselors, law enforcement, or other members of the law enforcement unit. The presence of a Confidential Record is to be noted on the student demographics pages of SASI under Confidential Record.

Level 1 Protocol: An assessment tool that guides the School Site Team as they complete the Level 1 Screening process.

Level 1 Recommended Treatment Providers List: provides a list of treatment and assessment providers who have some specialization with regard to sexual conduct.

Level 2 Flow Chart: Sexual Incident Response Team (Level 2 Specifics) – A visual detail of Level 2 process.

Level 2 Referral Guideline Flow Chart: A Visual representation of the recommended decision process for a Level 2 Assessment.

Level 2 Summary: Brief report summary of risk factors and management strategies identified through the level 2 process.

Parent Questionnaire – Level 1: A supplemental survey of questions intended as a guided interview to be completed by phone or in person with the parents or guardians of the student(s) being assessed through the Level 1 process. Is not to be given directly to the parents or guardians and is only to be used when the parents or guardians are unable to attend the Level 1 staffing. Questions correspond to Level 1 Protocol items and are a means of gathering as much information as possible.

Plan to Protect Targeted / Victimized Student: Documentation of safety planning for a student that has been targeted or victimized by another student.

Notification Letter: Written communication to legal guardians of threatened or victimized student. Oregon Statute requires phone notification within 12 hours and written notification within 24 hours. (See ORS. 339.250 and District Policy).

SALEM•KEIZER
PUBLIC SCHOOLS

1

Notification Log: Documentation of notification to the legal guardians of a threatened or victimized student. This form also provides a skeletal script for discussing the nature and circumstances of the threat and associated risk. Oregon Statute requires phone notification within 12 hours and written notification within 24 hours. (See ORS. 339.250 and District Policy).

Systems Flow Chart: Sexual Incident Response Committee (System Specific) – A visual representation of the entire student threat assessment system.

Teacher / Staff Questionnaire – Level 1: A supplemental survey of questions provided to teachers who are unable to attend the Level 1 staffing. Questions correspond to Level 1 Protocol items and are a means of gathering as much information as possible.

SALEM•KEIZER
PUBLIC SCHOOLS

GLOSSARY OF SIRC TERMS AND REFERENCES

504: Federal law requiring modifications for people with disabilities to access public agencies:

Access, Opportunity & Intent: Three factors most relevant in regard to safety planning. Access refers to the student's ability to engage with his/her object of sexual interest. Opportunity refers to the situations in which the student might initiate inappropriate sexual contact. Intent refers to the nature and intensity of the student's sexual interest. Ideally, safety planning should impact all three factors when possible. In the event that all three factors cannot be impacted, particular attention should be paid to strengthening the intensity of the interventions aimed at impacting the remaining factors.

ADA: Americans with Disabilities Act.

ADD: Attention Deficit Disorder.

Adjudication: This term is used for juveniles when the court finds them responsible for a crime, takes jurisdiction and places them on probation. Note: the adult equivalent would be "conviction". The term conviction is not used with juveniles…unless it is a Measure 11.

ASD: Autism Spectrum Disorder. (Special Ed. Identification.)

ATSA: Acronym for the Association for the Treatment of Sexual Abusers.

Affective Aggression / Reactive Aggression: Often used as synonymous terms, the two differ in the following ways. Affective aggression is an affectation of rage, power and or the capacity to inflict harm, often used to intimidate either before or during an attack. The attacker may be somewhat calculated in the effort, but is more often in a reactively aggressive position. Reactive aggression (impulsive, Impromptu) is without pre-meditation, planning plotting or specific targeting and is the result of either an imminent threat (real or perceived) or a sort of "last straw" loss of control resulting from an overwhelming situation. It can be affective and characterized by the emotions of anger and rage or be defensive and fearful. Either way, the goal is to eliminate the threat or the annoyance. Both aggressive strategies often occur in an emotional or highly aroused state and are responses to perceived challenge, threats, insults or other affronts. Both tend to be a matter of poor socialization or limited coping strategies.

Aspergers Syndrome: An Autism Spectrum Disorder. A sort of high functioning Autism. Is also considered a pervasive Development Disorder.

CCN: College Credit Now program at Chemeketa Community College.

CDS: Child Development Specialist (24J).

CST: Community Surveillance Team. (Juvenile Dept.)

DD: Developmental Disabilities.

DV: Domestic Violence.

DHS: Department of Human Services, previously known as SCF or Services to Children and Families.

DLC: Developmental Learning Center (Salem-Keizer School District program for low functioning developmentally delayed Students).

DTLC: Downtown Learning Center (Salem-Keizer School District program for GED and high school completion).

EAST: Early detection and treatment of psychosis and schizophrenia (first psychotic break or early indicators).

ECHS: Early College High School.

ED: Emotionally Disturbed (Special Education identification).

EGC: Emotional Growth Center. Self contained Special Ed. classroom for emotionally disturbed students.

ESD: Education Service District.

Evaluation: Used to indicate a mental health evaluation or psychological evaluation. Addresses the mental health, psychological issues as well as the behavioral issues of an individual.

Extensive Mutual Sexual Behaviors: Non-coercive, often developmentally non-normative, sexual behavior that occurs between two or more parties. Frequently noted among victims of physical abuse and abandonment, wherein the sexual behavior becomes a mechanism for relating to peers and self-soothing.

FSP: Family Support Program (Juvenile Department).

FSS: Family Support Specialist who works in Family support program at Juvenile department.

False Victimization: A false report of a crime or other incident that the actions taken as a result of the report will benefit the reporter. Characterized by attention seeking.

FAPA: Acronym for Family Abuse Prevention Act (Federal legislation on restraining orders). Used as a euphemism for a Restraining Order. (Also see RO.)

FERPA: Federal Education Rights Privacy Act.

Frotteurism: sexual paraphilia that involves rubbing one's genital area against an object or person.

Grooming: A process of identifying and engaging a victim in sexual activity that involves an imbalance of power, as well as coercion and manipulation with the intention to sexually exploit the victim.

SALEM•KEIZER
PUBLIC SCHOOLS

2

IDEA: Individuals with Disabilities Education Act.

IEP: Individual Education Plan.

IPS: In Program School.

Incarceration: Adults and/or parents that are in jail or prison.

Inhibitors: Those stabilizing factors that reduce the potential for individuals to engage in sexually inappropriate behavior. These include: religious beliefs, friends, family, employment, hobbies, pride, and dignity.

Intuition: Any quick insight, recognized immediately without a reasoning process; a belief arrived at unconsciously; -- often it is based on extensive experience of a subject.

Intervention: An action taken to decrease or stop sexually maladaptive behavior.

Johnson & Gil Typology for Sexually Acting Out Children: A method for categorizing children who act out sexually. Group 1: Normal Sexual Exploration. Group 2: Sexually Reactive Behaviors. Group 3: Extensive Mutual Sexual Behaviors. Group 4: Children Who Molest

LD: Learning disabled.

LSC: Life Skills Center (Salem-Keizer School District program for developmentally delayed students).

Level 1 Screening: Threat assessment, Firesetting, Suicide, and Sexual Incident screening done by a School Site Team consisting of an Administrator, Counselor/CDS, an SRO, a teacher who knows the student, and others as appropriate (parent, case manager if Special Ed. or 504, etc).

Level 2 Investigation: Threat assessment, Firesetting, Suicide, and Sexual Incident investigation done through the combined efforts of the Level 2 Team and School Site Team. Available if School Site Team determines, after conducting a Level 1 Investigation, that case needs further investigation, assessment and supervision.

Liaison Officer: Also referred to as (SRO) School Resource Officer.

MDT: Multi-disciplinary team.

Measure 11: Mandatory minimum sentencing crime.

MOU: Memorandum of Understanding.

MRDD: Mentally Retarded / Developmentally Disabled.

Mutually Inappropriate Sexual Behavior: Non-coercive sexual behavior that occurs between peers that although not illegal or necessarily maladaptive, is inappropriate given the context in which it occurs.

Normative Affection: Physical or verbal affection that is non-sexual and not disruptive

SALEM•KEIZER
PUBLIC SCHOOLS

Normative Sexual Development: sexual behavior that is consistent with developmental expectations and not pathological.

Non-normative Sexual Development: sexual behavior that is not developmentally consistent and which may be suggestive of maladaptive sexual development.

Opportunistic Sexual Intent: sexual intent that appears spontaneous, impulsive and/or unplanned.

Opportunistically Vigilant: Term referring to individuals who "watch the watchers" or individuals who otherwise give evidence that they are paying attention to supervisors for the purpose of taking advantage of decreased supervision.

OYA: Oregon Youth Authority.

PADTC: Polk Adolescent Day Treatment Center. (serves grades 6-12).

PCC: Psychiatric Crisis Center.

PDD: Pervasive Developmental Disorder characterized by abnormal social interaction and communication deficits.

PIRS: Prevention / Intervention Resource Specialist.

Playful Flirting: Fun, mutual, harmless, relationship enhancing, sexual behavior that is only a problem in that it may distract from school work.

POYAMA: Polk Yamhill Marion Counties day treatment center (serves grades K-6).

Premeditated Sexual Intent: sexual intent that appears to be planned and/or directed.

Protective Response: Initiated through Risk Management. An investigation and plan that addresses the physical vulnerability of a school, classroom, students and/or staff members. Used when a target has been identified through a threat.

Psychosexual Evaluation: A psychological evaluation typically conducted by a clinical psychologist or psychiatrist that examines psychological factors as they relate to sexual behavior. Typically, these evaluations address psychological/sexual development, psychopathology, personality characteristics, sexual preoccupations, safety planning, intent and risk assessment.

RAD: Reactive Attachment Disorder

Release Agreement: A written promise an arrestee agrees to upon release from custody pending trial on criminal charges. Also referred to as recognizance when the agreement is between the arrestee (Defendant) and the Court. Release agreements have general conditions such as a promise to appear in court as required, and may contain special conditions limiting the defendant's contacts, movements and behaviors.

SALEM•KEIZER
PUBLIC SCHOOLS

RO: Restraining Order. The acronym "TRO" is also sometimes used (Temporary Restraining Order) (See also FAPA).

Sexual Bullying: Aggressive, hurtful verbal or physical sexual behavior designed to intimidate or harm.

Sexual Harassment: Unwelcome and unwanted sexual words and behaviors/acts based on gender, being male/female, or sexual orientation.

Sexual Incident: Any verbal or physical (contact or non-contact) sexual behavior that occurs on school grounds, or during a school sponsored activity, or which otherwise impacts learning or student access to education. The following is an incomplete list of situations that constitute a sexual incident: sexual harassment, sexual bullying, exposing genitalia, mutually agreed to sexual touching, coerced or unwanted sexual touching, viewing/distributing pornography, sexting, etc.

Sexually Aggressive Behavior: Sexual behavior, including sexual harassment and sexual bullying, that although not illegal, demonstrates an imbalance of power, is harmful, and a violation of school policy.

Sexually Predatory Behavior: Coercive, developmentally non-normative sexual behavior that suggests the individual is preoccupied with identifying potential victims for sexual exploitation; may be typified by an imbalance of power between the participants. Individuals who engage in this behavior are typically remorseless and may use sexual behavior to vent unpleasant emotions. Oftentimes these individuals understand sex as an act of violence rather than intimacy.

Sexually Reactive Behaviors: sexual behaviors that are believed to stem from premature exposure to adult sexual behavior or sexual abuse. This behavior may appear somewhat compulsive and children who exhibit these behaviors may present as sexually preoccupied. Generally, the behavior is driven by anxiety about the premature exposure to adult sexual behavior, and is not predatory in nature.

SLC: Structured Learning Center (Salem-Keizer School District program for alternative education program).

SRO: School Resource Officer. Also referred to as Liaison Officer.

STAT: Mid-valley Student Threat Assessment Team. Members include Salem-Keizer School District, Marion County Sheriff's Department, Salem Police Department, Keizer Police Department, Marion County Court Security, Marion and Polk County Juvenile Departments, Oregon Youth Authority, Marion and Polk County Mental Health Departments, and Willamette Education Service District. The team conducts Level 2 assessment, assists with threat management strategies and explores resources.

SIRC: Mid-valley Sexual Incident Response Committee. Members include Salem-Keizer School District, Marion County Sheriff's Department, Salem Police Department, Keizer Police Department, Marion County Court Security, Marion and Polk County Juvenile Departments, Oregon Youth Authority, Marion and Polk County Mental Health Departments, and Willamette Education Service District. The team conducts Level 2 investigations, assists with threat management strategies and explores resources.

SALEM•KEIZER
PUBLIC SCHOOLS

Supervision Plan: A documented plan of modifications, interventions, and measures taken to reduce problems and circumstances that trigger, precipitate, or aggravate a dangerous situation. The Supervision Plan may also address long-term interventions.

Tarasoff : (Tarasoff Warning) (Tarasoff Principal) Reference to a University of California student who was stalked and killed by fellow student Prosenjit Poddar after he had discussed his intention to kill her with a University Health Service psychologist. Her family sued and the resulting court opinions formed the basis for general acceptance of the notion that treating professionals have a duty to protect known intended victims. (Tarasoff v. Regents, 17 Cal. 3d 425, 551 P.2d 334, 131 Cal. Rptr. 14 (1976).

TAT: Acronym for the Marion County, Threat Assessment Team.

Target: An individual, group or property identified as the focus of harm or damage in a threatening or dangerous situation.

Threat Assessment: The investigation of a threat made by an individual or group as well as an examination, survey and consideration of the behavior patterns, conditions, circumstances, and variables of danger in or surrounding an individual or group.

YCF: Youth Correctional Facility.

YST: Youth Services Team.

•••

This list was compiled by Rod Swinehart, Risk Management Consultant, Willamette Education Service District, John Van Dreal, School Psychologist, Salem-Keizer School District, and Wilson Kenney, School Psychologist, Salem-Keizer School District. It is not intended to be all-inclusive and to the definitions are intended to aid practioners not define terms for academics. Where known, credit is given to the authors. Where unknown, apologies are offered.

SALEM•KEIZER
PUBLIC SCHOOLS

Appendix F

Memorandum of Agreement
24J Sexual Incident Response Committee

This Agreement made and entered into as of the date set forth below, by and between: Salem-Keizer School District, Willamette ESD, Marion County Mental Health, Polk County Mental Health, Marion County Juvenile Department, Polk County Juvenile Department, Marion County Sheriff's Department, Salem Police Department, Keizer Police Department, Oregon Youth Authority, Marion County District Attorney's Office, and Polk County District Attorney's Office.

WHEREAS, all parties involved have agreed that controlling sexual misconduct is a community responsibility and that sharing resources through collaboration of community agencies is the best way to address it; and

WHEREAS, the team has developed a protocol that identifies and manages potentially dangerous sexual situations and circumstances in our schools and local community, as well as other communities in Marion and Polk Counties, and requires collaborative effort between agencies; and

WHEREAS, all parties are committed to improving services to adjudicated and pre-adjudicated youth identified by the 24J Sexual Incident Response Committee protocol, by sharing information, eliminating duplication of services, and coordinating efforts; and

WHEREAS, all parties mutually agree that sharing resources, where feasible, may result in improved coordination; and

WHEREAS, it is the understanding by all parties that certain roles in serving children and youth are required by law, and that these laws serve as the foundation for defining the role and responsibility of each participating agency; and

WHEREAS, all parties mutually agree that all obligations stated or implied in this agreement shall be interpreted in light of, and consistent with governing State and Federal laws;

NOW, THEREFORE in consideration of the following agreements, the parties agree to the following:

EACH OF THE PARTIES AGREE TO:

1. Meet on a weekly/bi-weekly basis to consult on cases that have been through the process. Each member agrees to participate in a weekly/bi-weekly meeting and be available for an emergency meeting if deemed necessary, or if unable to attend send a representative from their agency when feasible.

2. Keep the member's administrative authority fully advised of the team's activities in a manner satisfactory to the administrative authority and in a manner that accurately reflects the value that the team represents.

3. Attend and complete initial member training to be provided by the collaboration or through outside sources when available and feasible.

4. Continue to pursue additional training and knowledge in the area of threat assessment and management, and sexual misconduct to share this information with other team members.

5. Report immediately to the team any situations regarding perceived or potential conflicts of interest between the business of the team, the member, or with the member's organization.

6. Strictly comply with matters of confidentiality in a manner consistent with the members own agency policies and rules in dealing with confidential material. The parties to the agreement acknowledge that District 24J may disclose personally identifiable student information without prior written consent when the disclosure of that information relates to a court's or juvenile justice agency's ability to serve the needs of the student prior

SALEM•KEIZER
PUBLIC SCHOOLS

to adjudication under ORS Chapter 419C. The parties agree that they will not redisclose this information to any person or agency that is not a party to this agreement except as provided in ORS 336.187. Disclosure of personally identifiable information is authorized to the court, to the parties in this SIRC Agreement as a "juvenile justice agency", or to a person or organization providing direct services to the student on behalf of the SIRC.

7. Disclose information on adjudicated youth pursuant to FERPA rules and regulations.

8. Be sensitive to other participating agency issues, such as: jurisdiction, chains of command, agency business, and media and public perception.

9. While a member of the team, to not seek or accept personal gain resulting from either the training or knowledge inherent in being a team member.

ADMINISTRATIVE
This agreement shall be in effect beginning the date the agreement is signed by the parties and shall remain in effect until modified. It is expressly understood that any of the parties may terminate its participation in this agreement for whatever reason by giving sixty (60) days written notice to the other parties.

Modification of this agreement shall be made binding only by the consent of the majority of the parties. Any agreed upon modifications shall be made in writing and attached to this Agreement.

OTHER INTERAGENCY AGREEMENTS
All parties to this agreement acknowledge that this agreement does not preclude or preempt each of the agencies individually entering in to a separate agreement with one or more parties to this agreement. Such separate agreements shall not nullify the force and effect of this agreement. This agreement does not remove any other obligations imposed by laws to share information with other agencies.

Signed this date: _____

Agency / Organization: _____

Administrative Authority (Printed): _____

Administrative Authority (Signature): _____

Member's Name (Printed): _____

Member's Signature: _____

SALEM•KEIZER
PUBLIC SCHOOLS

SIGN IN SHEET

Sexual Incident Response Committee

Date: _____

Student Name:_____School: _____

I have read, understood, and will abide
By the Confidentiality Agreement of SIRC.

Please PRINT Your Name
Thank you.....

~ SIRC ~
SEXUAL INCIDENT RESPONSE COMMITTEE
SIRC Does Not Case Manage.
SIRC is a Consultation Team that Investigates Incidents of Sexual Misconduct and
Assists Case Managers with Threat Management and Identification of Resources.

CONFIDENTIALITY AGREEMENT FOR SIRC

While staffing incidents of sexual misconduct through the SIRC process, the following rules
apply:

1. The confidentiality policies of your agency / organization apply.

2. You are responsible for any material (hard copy, documents, reports, etc.) that you
   present and its dissemination and retrieval after presentation.

3. You are responsible for the confidentiality (see #1) of any documents collected through
   staffing. You have agreed not to redisclose personally identifiable information about
   students obtained during the SIRC process except as pursuant to ORS 336.187 and the
   Memorandum of Agreement.

4. As circumstances change, cases may be restaffed by SIRC at the request of case
   managers.

5. I will immediately declare any potential conflict of interest that I discover, regarding the
   student of focus, with members present or agencies represented.

_____   _____   _____
Sign Name   **Title/Location**   **Date**

                              _____
                                     PRINT Name

SIRC Confidentiality Agreement

SALEM•KEIZER
PUBLIC SCHOOLS

References

Dunklin, R. (2017). Sex assaults in high school sports minimized as 'hazing.' Retrieved from https://www.ap.org/explore/schoolhouse-sex-assault/sex-assaults-in-high-school-sports-minimized-as-hazing.html.

Dunklin, R., & Schmall, E. (2017). Kindergarteners among youngest schoolhouse assault victims. Retrieved from https://www.ap.org/explore/schoolhouse-sex-assault/kindergarteners-among-youngest-schoolhouse-assault-victims.html.

Hanson, K., Bourgon, G., Helmus, L., & Hodgson, S. (2009). *A meta-analysis of the effectiveness of treatment for sexual offenders: Risk, need, and responsivity.* Ottawa, Canada: Public Safety Canada.

Letourneau, E., & Bourdin, C. (2008). The effective treatment of juveniles who sexually offend: An ethical imperative. *Ethics & Behavior, 18*(2/3), 286–306.

Letourneau, E., Henggeler, S., Borduin, C., Schewe, P., McCart, M., Chapman, J., et al. (2009). Multisystemic therapy for juvenile sexual offenders: 1-year results from a randomized effectiveness trial. *Journal of Family Psychology, 23*(1), 89–102.

Lhamon, C. E. (2015). Questions and answers on Title IX and sexual violence. U.S. Department of Education, Office for Civil Rights. Retrieved from https://www2.ed.gov/about/offices/list/ocr/docs/qa-201404-title-ix.pdf.

Linderman, J. (2017). Clash over middle-school sex assaults: Did they happen? Retrieved from https://www.ap.org/explore/schoolhouse-sex-assault/clash-over-middle-school-sex-assaults-did-they-happen.html.

McDowell, R., Dunklin, R., Schmall, E., & Pritchard, J. (2017). Hidden horror of school sex assaults revealed by AP. Retrieved from https://www.ap.org/explore/schoolhouse-sex-assault/hidden-horror-of-school-sex-assaults-revealed-by-ap.html.

O'Banion, L. K. (2018). Campus sexual assault and (In)justice: An inquiry into campus grievance professionals' roles, responsibilities, and perspectives of justice. *Dissertations and Theses.* Paper 4407. https://pdxscholar.library.pdx.edu/open_access_etds/4407. doi:10.15760/etd.6291.

Office of Civil Rights (OCR). (2001). *Revised sexual harassment guidance: Harassment of students by school employees, other students, or third parties.* Washington DC: U.S. Department of Education. Retrieved from https://www2.ed.gov/about/offices/list/ocr/docs/shguide.pdf.

Office of Civil Rights (OCR). (September, 2017). *Q&A on campus sexual misconduct.* Washington DC: U.S. Department of Education. Retrieved from https://ww w2.ed.gov/about/offices/list/ocr/docs/qa-title-ix-201709.pdf.

Pritchard, J., & Dunklin R. (2017). Schools face vexing test: Which kids will sexually attack? Retrieved from https://www.ap.org/explore/schoolhouse-sex-assault/scho ols-face-vexing-test-which-kids-will-sexually-attack.html.

Pritchard, J., Flaccus, G., & Dunklin R. (2017). Students, some schools take on sexual assault. Retrieved from https://www.ap.org/explore/schoolhouse-sex-assault/stud ents-some-schools-take-on-sexual-assault.html.

Przybylski, R. (2014). Chapter 5: Effectiveness of treatment for juveniles who sexually offend. Retrieved from https://www.smart.gov/SOMAPI/sec2/ch5tre atment.html.

Reitzel, L. R., & Carbonell, J. L. (2006). The effectiveness of sexual offender treatment for juveniles as measured by recidivism: A meta-analysis. *Sexual Abuse: Journal of Research and Treatment, 18*(4), 401–421. doi:10.1007/s11194-006-9031-2.

Rosner, R. (2003). *Principals and practice of forensic psychiatry.* Boca Raton, FL: Taylor & Francis Group.

Schmall, E., & Dunklin, R. (2017). School sex complaints to federal agency rise – and languish. Retrieved from https://www.ap.org/explore/schoolhouse-sex-assault/school-sex-complaints-to-federal-agency-rise-and-languish.html.

Schmucker, M., & Lösel, F. (2008). Does sexual offender treatment work? A systemic review of outcome evaluations. *Psicothema, 20*(1), 10–19.

Smith, M. (2017). Students sexually abused at school face lengthy legal fights. Retrieved from https://www.ap.org/explore/schoolhouse-sex-assault/students-sexually-abused-at-school-face-lengthy-legal-fights.html.

TITLE IX OF THE EDUCATION AMENDMENTS
OF 1972, 20 U.S.CODE §1681 ET SEQ.

34 C.F.R. Part 106- Nondiscrimiation on the Basis of Sex in Education Programs or Activities Receiving Federal Financial Assistance.

Franklin v. Gwinnet County Public Schools, 503 U.S. 60 (1992).

Gebser v. Lago Vista Indep. School, 524 U.S. 274 (1998).

Davis V. Monroe County Bd. of Educ., 526 U.S. 629 (1999).

Office of Civil Rights Dear Colleague letter January 2001 (Revised Sexual Harassment Guidance: Harassment of Students by School Employees, Other Students, or Third Parties).

Office of Civil Rights Dear Colleague letter April 2011 (Sexual Violence (Withdrawn September 2017)).

Office of Civil Rights Dear Colleague letter April 2014 (Questions and Answers about Title IX and Sexual Violence (April 2014) (Withdrawn September 2017)).

Office of Civil Rights Dear Colleague letter February 2017 (Withdrawing Title IX Guidance on Transgender Students).

Office of Civil Rights Dear Colleague letter September 2017 (Withdrawing Guidance on Sexual Violence).

Office of Civil Rights Q&A on Campus Sexual Misconduct September 2017.

About the Author

J. Wilson Kenney received his doctorate in Clinical Psychology from the University of Utah in 2007. Since then, he has worked as a school psychologist, and served as clinical director for a residential, outpatient, and proctor-care, sex offender treatment facility. Currently, Wilson provides behavioral and threat mitigation consultation to school districts, and forensic assessment through the Center for Integrated Intervention, and threat-of-harm consultation to private organizations as a consulting psychologist for Foresight Security Consulting. Wilson's areas of specialization include personality disorder, problematic sexual behavior, threat assessment, and forensic assessment. Wilson is a licensed psychologist and certified forensic evaluator. He currently serves on the Commission on Judicial Fitness & Disability, and he previously served on the Review Panel for Forensic Evaluators.

Made in the USA
Monee, IL
08 November 2022

17326015R00125